I'VE HEARD
THE VULTURES
SINGING

I'VE HEARD THE VULTURES SINGING

Field Notes on Poetry, Illness, and Nature

Lucia Perillo

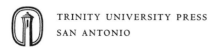

TRINITY UNIVERSITY PRESS
SAN ANTONIO

Published by Trinity University Press
San Antonio, Texas 78212

Jacket design by Erin Kirk New
Book design by BookMatters, Berkeley

⊗ The paper used in this publication meets the minimum
requirements of the American National Standard for
Information Sciences—Permanence of Paper for Printed
Library Materials, ANSI Z39.48-1992.

Library of Congress Cataloging-in-Publication Data

Perillo, Lucia Maria, 1958–
    I've heard the vultures singing : field notes on poetry,
illness, and nature / Lucia Perillo.
        p. cm.
    Summary: "Poet Lucia Perillo, who once worked as
a park ranger and was diagnosed with multiple sclerosis
in her thirties, confronts the ironies of going from an
outdoors person to someone who can no longer walk.
Among other topics, these essays explore how poetry
provides an alternative means of accessing nature"—
Provided by publisher.
    ISBN-13: 978-1-59534-031-3 (hardcover : alk. paper)
    ISBN-10: 1-59534-031-9 (hardcover : alk. paper) 1. Perillo,
Lucia Maria, 1958– 2. Poets, American—20th century—
Biography. I. Title.
    PS3566.E69146Z46   2007
    814'.54—dc22   2007003686

11 10 09 08 07 C 5 4 3 2 1

For my mother

Everything in nature is lyrical in its ideal essence,
tragic in its fate, and comic in its existence.

GEORGE SANTAYANA

CONTENTS

ACKNOWLEDGMENTS

These essays first appeared, in earlier drafts, in the following books and journals: *American Poetry Review, Georgia Review, Michigan Quarterly Review, Northwest Review, poemmemoirstory, River Styx, Short Takes: Brief Encounters with Contemporary Nonfiction,* and *Tin House.* I would like to thank the editors of those publications for their scrupulous attention to my prose, and thanks also to the other people who looked at these essays as I thought my way through them: Ed Brunner, Scott Chambers, Sandra Fisher, Angus Heriot, Dorianne Laux, Maria McLeod, Marva Nelson, Suzanne Paola, James Rudy, Ben Sonnenberg. Steve Howie is the person to be either thanked or blamed for first suggesting to me that my life was interesting when I never would have thought it so.

A Glimpse

Right now, a tiger named Andrea who lives in the Portland Zoo is dying of cancer in her uterus. The zookeepers might have caught the disease earlier if only she hadn't kept it hidden, but animals are programmed not to give away their symptoms lest their predators take notice and begin the chase. There is a biological imperative that drives us not to show any traces of our pains, not to reveal any clues about our grip on existence having weakened. In the wild, the lame are quickly eaten, an efficient solution to the problem of disease, without even a need for cleaning up, thanks to the carrion-eaters and then the microbes.

It's probably because I studied wildlife biology in college that my mind tends to drift in the direction of wondering what my life would be like if I were a wild animal. As a young woman, I worked as a ranger in a variety of wildernesses, and I was vain about having a body that could paddle me across the sea or climb me to the top of mountains without complaint except sometimes a little twinkling in the balls of my feet. When these sensations became more electrical, when the fog out of which I'd always built my daydreams was pierced at odd moments by a fork of lightning, I found myself lying for half an hour inside a machine that clanged as if it were being pounded by a hammer. Since this imaging technology had only recently become available and the hospital in my town did not yet own such a machine, I'd entered one that pulled into town on a tractor-trailer, like the circus. So as not to blur the image, the technician warned me not to flinch.

A week later the photographic sheets were developed, revealing many cross-sections of my brain, laid out in columns and rows that had been marked with arrows, which pointed to white spots that the neurologist said indicated damage. That was when he named the disease, *my* disease as we say, as if having a disease conferred a kind of ownership, which would imply some degree of control. The name is made of syllables that are not suited to poetry. *Leukemia, Lupus, Spanish influenza*: any of these I could maybe do something with. But *multiple sclerosis* is just not workable from a poet's point of view. In addition to that, it frightened me. For years I could not bear to see the word *multiple* printed anywhere, or my bones would dissolve and my lungs would refuse to be inflated.

The day after the doctor told me what had gone wrong with my body, I went skiing alone on Mount Rainier, where just a few months before I'd worked as a back-country ranger and had mastered the art of making those delicate telemark turns that require dropping to one knee like a man proposing with a ring. The new snow was thick and wet, what people call Cascade Concrete, and avalanche warnings had been posted at the ranger station. I had a dramatic idea about dying in an avalanche as I skied down the saddle between two peaks in the Tatoosh Range. To be packed like a supermarket fish in snow—I wanted to ride out of the world that way, and I drove home feeling a little disappointed about not being dead (but exhilarated, too, about having outwitted my bad number).

That last sentence included the kind of sentiment (*I was a little disappointed about not being dead*) that comes off as anti-social, living as we do in an age that mandates soldiering onward in the face of illness. The sick tiger walks the length of the bars in her cage in the zoo as if nothing's wrong, and we humans ask each other how we're doing every day; as a chorus of millions chants, *Fine*. It's as if we have transposed the animal imperative not to expose our weaknesses, from body-language into words.

But to resist enlisting as a brave soldier in the battle against one's illness—to choose instead burial by avalanche!—seems to me to be a typically human and honest response (or the honest response of one typical sort of human) to the news that one's life might be marked by faster-than-normal physical decay. The doctor's operative word was *might*, and the uncertainty was what I found unbearable in those early days when I hunted for a story or a portent in any form—tarot cards or tea leaves—to tell me about my future.

The only story I found useful was one by Jorge Luis Borges in which he describes the infinite Library of Babel. It's a place that turns some men into murderers and drives others mad as each one searches for his own Book of Vindications, which will tell him the story of his death at the same time as it forgives him of his wrongs. But the infinite number of books in this library makes the hunt futile. There are too many books to search through. I bring up Borges's story by way of saying that anyone looking to find his or her body here should be forewarned that this particular ride has already been taken.

In fact, my version of my illness has left me—slowly, over the course of twenty years—ever more physically compromised, and I have felt deficient of both willpower and spiritual vigor in being unable to control the slip and swoop and skid. To speak of this does not seem *seemly* because our tribe likes to hear stories of the body rising; perhaps this, too, is a remnant of that old necessity to not lure the wolves.

Foolishly, then, I leave this record of my recent years, of my life indoors and out. At times I think I'm barely living; I can hear the air being stirred by the vultures that circle overhead, and then *zing*—an eagle will battle a seagull over a stickleback, right in town beside the abandoned fried-chicken restaurant. Then my presence is confirmed, in the same stroke as the world says: *you are not done here yet*.

The painter Willem de Kooning famously called himself *a slipping glimpser*, slipping into the glimpse—slipping toward the image—that he would then arrest in paint. I spend much of my time trying to write poems about what I can single out from my own slipping, which is difficult because when you're slipping you tend to keep your eyes trained on your feet to keep from crashing; it's hard to lift your eyes so that the world can be attended to. Easy to forget, the world is still occurring outside the drama of the self, and the poem of the self is going to be limited unless the world can enter in. The down-tug of disease also tends to turn the glimpse into a blur, because the observer is in constant motion. How to capture the glimpse, to freeze it and make it legible? Or should the glimpse be captured in a manner that somehow incorporates the blur, the way that de Kooning's paintings are all swirl and motion?

There's also the dilemma that whatever I say or write today will be outdated tomorrow, because by then I will have slipped to a different place, most likely at a lower elevation, at least from the point of view of the flesh. If there's any consolation to be taken in such a life, the slipping life, it may be in the sheer speed and whooshing of its passage. At least it is not ordinary, and I can take heart in the oddness of my path, even though it did not lead me to the kind of wilderness I expected. Funny how I did end up inside the avalanche after all, not dead. And I could say there is a peculiar glamour in being stuffed with all these glittering crystals, but I'm not crazy enough to make that claim.

KNOWLEDGE GAME: *Gulls*

Downtown, behind an empty warehouse and the sewage plant, Puget Sound sticks a thumb into the mouth of Moxlie Creek. This is one place I go to watch seabirds—now that I can't walk, I can't be too picky about what incarnation of nature I'll accept. I've been forced to gerrymander my definition of the wilderness, if I'm to have any wilderness at all. Often this means staring at the mud that is the bottom of the bay, where gulls battle over scraps of dead sea life while the water is retracted elsewhere by the tide.

Swantown is the historical name of this place, though *Costa del Bum* is what I call it—homeless men lounge here in their winter parkas, even when the sun is blazing. The sun's appearance will cause businessmen and joggers to lie down here too, on this fingernail-paring's worth of grass that must be mowed by God; at least I've never seen anyone else take care of it. The lions and lambs, the yuppies and hobos, like a scene from a Jehovah's Witness pamphlet.

The only drawback is the musky rotting smell, which

you'll get used to soon enough—and when you acclimate, the odor will grow close to being sweet.

The smell gets worse when the water disappears, and it eases up when the water reappears again a half-day later. Meanwhile the gulls gather on the nearby warehouse's rounded quonset roof, standing there like compliant citizens waiting on the platform for a train. Sometimes they'll erupt into a round of violent squawks, but just as suddenly their anger's gone, the way the bay goes a little crazy when a rock's thrown into it but soon grows calm again.

To fill the space of body-motion, I play knowledge games that substitute for the physical ones I've lost. I play my games to trick myself into believing that the simple act of walking isn't what I miss most of all (a grief that might be too obvious to have to state, though I always have to remind myself that there do exist in this world people like my father—well, he doesn't exist anymore, except in my memory, where he is still a man who parks with an outlaw's recklessness in order to be not more than a few steps away from whatever doorway he's about to enter. When I took him to national parks, he sat in the car and waited for me to return from circuiting the half-mile nature trail. The irony that's been awarded to him posthumously is that his tombstone can't be seen from the road.)

The point of these knowledge games is to be outdoors, focused on something that lies outside my own body, which happens to be not walking but wheeling along. I figure I might as well pick something difficult to be the object of the knowledge game, to consume a lot of mental energy as though this were equivalent to the calorie-burning of jogging. Hence the attraction of gulls, whose identification is near impossible.

Field Note from 9/26

I'm looking at Costa del Bum from across the bay at Priest Point Park, where my friends have encouraged me to climb down from the scooter and lie on the mud so I can feel it against my spine, poor spine that rarely gets a chance to straighten. The only birds on the water are the gulls, and my line of sight is flush with them . . . but I've forgotten the field guide, which sets my project back from the start.

My project being: to give each gull a name.

Instead, I start by watching their beaks open when they lunge toward one another, their tongues flickering like the tongues of snakes. Their feathers look thick and solid, a white hide from which it would be hard to draw blood.

Because I want to get a good look at them, we lay down near the water's edge, and the tide that was low when we arrived is soon lapping at my feet. Then it turns out that my friends have overestimated both their strength and mine, and when they have trouble erecting me, we have to call over a guy who's been watching us, looking perplexed. He's hanging back from the rest of his group of kids and adults who are wading.

"I wouldn't go in that water. That water's nasty," he says, gesturing with his beer can.

"No, it is beautiful—what's wrong with it?"

"All that dead stuff," he says, tottering as he lifts me.

Beyond being a knowledge game, this gull-watching is also part of a self-improvement program I've launched—trying to train myself not to overlook the common thing. *Why does the rare thing arouse more interest? Why doesn't a gull compel anybody like an eagle would?* One answer could be that this phenomenon is a by-product of the tendency toward procrastination that is inherent in human nature. We assume the common things will always be here, so we tell ourselves we'll deal with them another day.

Whereas if an eagle soars by, which is not so unlikely at a place like Costa del Bum (part of a small city that happens to contain some eagle habitat), we'll feel obligated to memorize whatever anecdote it creates for future retelling, particularly if it performs a dramatic, violent feat. We build our conversation from this game of one-upmanship:

"I saw an eagle swoop over the backyard while I was mowing the lawn."

"One snatched a salmon off my barbecue."

"Oh, I have a good friend who's an eagle." Et cetera.

Gulls, on the other hand, possess less narrative value—it can be tough to cull a good story from their fitful scavenging. Raymond Carver's poem "Eagles" tells of sautéing a ling cod that an eagle has dropped: consuming this fish makes the narrator feel connected with "an older, fiercer order of things." Eating something dropped by a gull, on the other hand, would not inspire this kind of noble sentiment—because the dropped thing would most likely be trash.

Field Note from 11/6

I've scoped these gulls out as herring gulls, distinguishable by their pink legs. "Abundant, widespread, increasing" says the bird book, "the most common large gull over most of North America." So I take that name and run.

When I'm thinking about birds, I think of Emily Dickinson, who wrote so many bird poems that birds could be called her signature subjects (well, birds and also the shadow-version of their restless movement, which is the stock-stillness of death). The handy thing about birds is that you can spy them from your window even if you never leave your house, as gradually became the case with Dickinson, famous for her reclusiveness. A bit of luck that she was drawn to birds. A graver tragedy would be for her to have been a tidepool enthusiast, because it's hard to imagine the kind of storm that would send a hermit crab flying by.

In fact, Emily Dickinson didn't write any poems about gulls—the only connection I'm making is that she, too, lived under circumstances that limited what parts of nature she could access. And though the location of her fieldwork was restricted (maybe her backyard wasn't ever passed over by the inverted droopy W's of gulls), she chose to retain nature for subject matter, instead of turning away from it, which would have been the easier course of action.

"The Robin's my Criterion for Tune— / Because I grow— where Robins do— / But, were I Cuckoo born— / I'd swear by him— " Dickinson wrote, explicitly stating her satisfaction with using whatever nature is at hand. It takes courage to spend time considering nature when your life is circumscribed, because this means considering what you have lost.

Dickinson's most famous bird poem was written in 1861, during a five-year period of feverish production. It opens:

"Hope" is the thing with feathers—
That perches in the soul—
And sings the tune without the words—
And never stops—at all—

Because I'd learned this poem's first line out of context, I took it to mean that birds in general were hopeful things. But when you see the whole poem you understand it's the other way around: the idea of "Hope" is being made into a bird. (And why the quotes? Is it because *Hope* is being used as shorthand for a more complicated psychic brew, the way people will hold up two fingers of each hand like hooks to scratch the air, a gesture that is supposed to encapsulate an idea already circulating in the culture at large?)

When I worked as a naturalist on San Francisco Bay, birds freaked me out a little. What I found frightening was the degree to which the plumage functions as a cloak that keeps you from seeing the bird as it really is. You'd see the gull with its thick hide shining and think it was a perfect, sturdy thing. But then a dead gull would turn up in one of the salt ponds that comprised the refuge. And you'd realize that, underneath the feathers, a bird is little more than a skeleton with a beating heart inside. Their beauty is an artifact, created by their constant preening. They spend the bulk of their hours on what could seem like narcissistic self-concern because grooming keeps them from freezing or drowning or getting parasitized or eaten.

A different poet foolishly equated beauty with truth, but in the case of gulls beauty equals survival.

Field Note from 11/29

I'm leapfrogging a pair of young men at the lake in the center of town, advancing past them and being advanced when I stop to look through my binoculars. Lots of ducks, but the gulls too far out to see. I see a beaver noodling around just a few yards from my feet, and when the men advance toward me I whisper: Look.

(Such self-importance attached to being the one who spots the animal, to being the one who wins the contest of perception. I'm a little embarrassed when I find myself playing this game.)

These men, I realize, are an autistic man and his caregiver walking on a sunny day. The caregiver points his caregiven toward the beaver, but the autistic man, in his blue windbreaker, keeps turning to look at me. On my cart, with its basket full of books and pens, I'm more interesting to him than any wild creature. Or maybe I am a wild creature—this idea appeals to me.

Only it turns out that I am wrong about this beaver, who is in fact a nutria, a South American rodent introduced for its fur, thirteen of them imported to Louisiana by the hot sauce baron McIlhenny in 1937. Now they've chewed their way to the Northwest—"eat outs" are what you call areas of infestation where the marsh grasses are completely grazed. The state of Louisiana is trying to solve the problem by popularizing them as a recipe ingredient. Most of the recipes call for hot sauce, I note.

Invasive swamp rat, destroyer of wetlands, a trash animal like the gull. How quickly the mind swivels in response to what it learns.

Dickinson equated birds with time's passage because they migrate. Their recurrences are a reminder that another year has passed, that death has taken a step closer.

> I dreaded that first Robin, so,
> But He is mastered, now,
> I'm some accustomed to Him grown
> He hurts a little, though—

And because they leave, she sees them also as the embodiments of grief:

'Tis not that Dying hurts us so—
'Tis Living—hurts us more—
But Dying—is a different way—
A Kind behind the Door—

The Southern Custom—of the Bird—
That ere the Frosts are due—
Accepts a better Latitude—
We—are the Birds—that stay.

Staying is hard, the staying is work, because of the sorrow that comes from being abandoned by the dead. Migration became a code, a shorthand for the way that many of her friends died while Dickinson kept on living.

Gulls do not abandon us, though—they always seem to be loitering in our midst. Not that death doesn't come as a parcel with their company: you can't stare for too long at the water's edge before some part of a dead gull comes washing up, the primary feathers ragged around the translucent spike of the white shaft. There's something terrible about it—because the living bird looks so pristine—and one's first impulse is to turn away from the sodden feather barbs, turned into scraggly threads. How not to be repulsed by the wet gray meat of the breast?

But I'm trying to teach myself not to be squeamish when it comes to looking, looking being one thing I can still do. This is how my life is shaped these days, by process of elimination: I do what I can still do. Somehow it's always interesting, at least so far.

Field Note from 12/3

A pair of hooded mergansers is dabbling at something below the surface, and the gulls keep swooping, trying to drive them off. As soon as the ducks find another spot to dabble, the gulls want it too—and so they move around the bay off Costa del Bum like checkers.

The male hooded merganser is my favorite bird, what with its spectacular freakish head, which looks like nothing special until the crest that slumps off the back of the head lifts up and spreads out like a fan. The male's head is black, with a white patch that widens behind his eye when the crest is raised.

A jogger approaches, then holds up, running in place so he can ask what I'm looking at. "Oh, just gulls," I say. It's not even worth attempting to feel self-important when squaring off against a guy who's wearing Lycra tights. He wins—he's the superior being. Defeated, I shrivel up and will not speak.

I was married off the coast of Costa del Bum, on an old wooden boat called *The Lotus*. At the little ceremony, which seems so ridiculous in retrospect, we quoted Archibald Mac-Leish: "We say that *Amor vincit omnia* but in truth love conquers nothing—certainly not death—certainly not chance. What love does is to arm. It arms the worth of life in spite of life." This is a gull kind of statement—that life is brutal, that you have to approach it with suspicion and a sharp hooked beak. Archibald MacLeish is long dead and maybe not held in anyone's esteem as a poet anymore, but the quote is one thing I retain from the wedding ceremony that I'm not embarrassed about, because it turned out to suit my life so well.

Jim remembers sweeping the dock to get rid of the bird shit and the broken shells that the gulls had dropped, and so the first picture that I painted, of the gulls as trash-eaters, was incomplete. Of course they eat mollusks, and they also eat chicks that stray—my old ornithology textbook says this cannibalization accounts for as much as 70 percent of the mortality of their young. If I were a gull, my neighbors would have already finished me off.

"But you are not a gull," Jim reminds me. That old admonishment again.

Phone Machine, 1/11

Gordon, the Audubon volunteer, leaves a message in response to my inquiry. He gives me web addresses where I can find the bird checklist from the nearby wildlife refuge, as well as the tally from last year's Christmas Bird Count. It turns out I've been completely wrong: there are no herring gulls on the bird count, and the wildlife refuge lists them as only a rare visitor here in winter.

Like most people, I apportion my interest in the natural world according to formulae I'm not consciously aware of, formulae in which the population size of a creature has an inverse relation to that creature's hold on my imagination. What I mean is: rare = good (though the many poems written to the common crow are an exception, probably because they appeal to us in a libidinous way—the ancient Greeks used the phrase *going to the crows* where we would say *going to the devil*).

Pretty does not necessarily equal good. There is a great deal of beauty in the Canada goose's face, the bird that's been rounded up and gassed at Costa del Bum because it soiled all the Jehovah's-Witness-pamphlet grass. I still see gangs of lazy mallards there, the males with their stunning green heads. But I skip on, as soon as I've got the name— *there's a mallard, what next? And, as soon as I've found that bird, what next?*

Here are all the birds whose sightings numbered over a thousand on the Christmas Bird Count:

Canada Goose	2,358
American Widgeon	5,546
Mallard	2,281
Northern Pintail	1,078
Surf Scoter	2,120
Bufflehead	2,346
Dunlin	2,356
Glaucous-winged Gull	1,824
Glaucous-winged Gull × Western Gull (hybrid)	1,318

Crow	2,050
Golden Crowned Kinglet	1,173
American Robin	1,414
European Starling	5,307
Dark-eyed (Oregon) Junco	1,382
Red-winged Blackbird	1,353
Pine Siskin	3,515

What stumps me about myself is how—even now, midway through a season of trying to prick up my powers of attention—how oblivious I am. To kinglets, siskins, widgeons: to all the common birds I've missed.

Conversation with Gordon the Audubon Guy, 1/17

Me: Okay. I found the checklist and figured out that in all likelihood the big gulls I'm seeing are either glaucous-winged gulls or glaucous-winged/western hybrids, but I'm not sure how people are making this distinction. I think the hybrids are darker on the wing edge? And the herring gulls look pretty similar, but now I see that the others have a white spot visible on the mantle when the bird is sitting, have I got that right? And there are two other gulls that are common, but from the book I can tell they're smaller, the mew gull and the ring-billed and the ring on the bill of the mew is a little less pronounced, but is there a trick to telling the size differential if you don't have the big gull and the little one side by side?

When I finally stop talking, Gordon answers: Here's where you're getting over my head.

Maybe the problem with gulls stems from the fact that they have very little mythic dimension. In my book of Indian legends from the Pacific Northwest, there's no mention of them. The Greeks and the Romans give them short shrift when compared with glamour-birds like nightingales. In his play *The Birds*, Aristophanes makes just one brief mention of the gull, linking it to Hercules, who is made out to be a foolish glutton.

In this coastal town the gulls soar everywhere, crapping on our cars. We too associate them with gluttony, because of the way they raid the dumpsters at the fast-food joints, and even their genus name, *Larus*, comes from a Latin word that means "ravenous seabird."

When the salmon are running, gulls take up residence in the woods, where they feed on salmon carcasses. And here they become especially frightening because they are so far out of their shoreline context; instead, they flap and squawk between the limbs of cedars. They swoop past at such low altitude that you can stare into their eyes without lifting up your head. How frightening to see the ravenous bird from such an unaccustomed angle, at such an unaccustomed proximity, in such an unaccustomed place.

Field Note from 1/18

The gulls are gathered on the warehouse roof, but, before I can circumnavigate the crotch of the bay, the shadows start to lie flat on the ground. Suddenly, the gulls fly off to a spot on the other side of the bay—where I just came from—that's still sunlit. By the time I cross back over, all I can see are silhouettes. Black shapes all identical.

Late in her life, Dickinson revisited the subject of hope in poems that echo her famous early poem. "Hope is a strange invention— / A patent of the Heart"—a stiffer, more mechanical depiction than the hope she once deposited in the breast. A short while later comes a poem in which "Hope is a subtle Glutton" who "feeds upon the fair." Now hope is ravenous, like the gulls, and we are being eaten alive, as in my fantasy where I say: *take me, take me*. It's the fantasy of a sudden, cut-off end.

When Gordon the Audubon guy gives me the e-mail address of Bill—who's supposed to be the go-to guy on bird identification in this town—the electronic ether never answers. Then I find on my shelf an old book from the 1950s called *Our Amazing Birds: Little Known Facts about Their Private Lives*. There's a glitch in the printing, though, that leaves the page on gulls a blank. The strange synchronicities start to build, spreading to Emily Dickinson even. One of her last bird poems goes:

> If I should see a single bird
> [*remaining text unknown*]

Note how, even with the missing line, the couplet sustains Dickinson's characteristic 4 beat/3 beat meter.

Field Note from 1/24

I've tracked down a book about the Swantown birds, produced from several years of censuses made by a local ornithologist who restricted his counts to "birds floating or just taking flight from the water, except gulls" on the grounds that identifying the gulls would "suck up too much time."

Here I am, watching them float in the bay and stand on the pilings, and I think I've nailed down the basics. Large gull with pink legs, you make your call based on the darkness of the wings. If the field marks are at odds, call it a hybrid. Call the smaller gulls mews unless you see a distinct ring around their bills. Forget the juveniles because you'll never get them straight.

But at least half the gulls are drab brown juveniles. With any luck, I can guess the names of maybe half the rest. This means my best chance of success is 1 in 4. Probable outcome: 75 percent failure. I have to live with that.

Four years after we got married, Jim and I saw *The Lotus* leaking oil one day when we paddled by in our kayak. It was slowly sinking, and we helped the Department of Ecology set up a ring of yellow buoys around it. This is the kind of occurrence that seems ripe for metaphor—the wedding boat sinking, the two of us saving the environment from contamination. *The Lotus* was eventually sold, then vanished—another cut-off end.

Field Note from 2/1

I've got a loaf of dark rye bread that's been sitting on
the kitchen counter with a 1/11 expiration date, and I'm
at Costa del Bum, tearing the slices into scraps. Half
the gulls float in the water and half sit on the streetlamps.
At first they ignore the scraps I throw until the crows
start moving in, which cues the gulls to my attempt to
lure them. Then it's just a matter of continuing to fling
my bits and crusts, and when I roll backward a horde
of gulls, in their white helmets, crowds the cinder path.
Suddenly, I can see how the situation could become
dangerous if they decided to challenge me for the bread.

Clear, though, are their gradations of colors, the fair
wings and darker ones, the mismatched tails of the hybrids.
I don't even need binoculars to discern the spots on their
beaks. The ashy juveniles come closest, maybe a sign of
their stupidity. Further back, the adults cry like squeaky
hinges. They all scare off when two women come along
with a dog, who craps unabashedly on the grass where I'd
lured my throng, and the women move on without picking
up their remnant.

Times like this, I curse the human race.

But when the dog is gone, the gulls assemble again,
feinting toward each other with their yellow beaks and
shivering tongues. How you make gulls compelling, I
discover, is by summoning them. No doubt bread is bad
for a wild animal's digestive system—I once worked for
the U.S. Fish & Wildlife Service, I know this—and I

shouldn't be encouraging these gulls in more beggarly
habits than they already own. But any rush of power is
amplified to a person who can't help feeling powerless,
and I can't resist convening them, my hundred Roman
citizens. Whose names at last I think I know, though
I am probably wrong.

Definition of Terms

Sometimes I call myself *cripple*, a word that comes from the Old English *creopan*, meaning "to go bent down." So, etymologically, cripples are creepy. Our bodies house the worst sort of luck, and I would bet that most people are afraid to see themselves in the bent form's mirror—as if bad body-luck were contagious and traveled via the eye-beams, a belief that seems somehow intuitively logical. Even though my own animal fortune has packed its bags and headed south, I'm not immune to a hitch in my swallow whenever I cross paths with the likes of me.

As a member of the population to which the word applies, though, I'm given some latitude in my use of *cripple* as an aggressive form of self-description. In doing so I may intend to suggest that I have become hardened to its connotations, or that I am a realist about my body's state, or that I am using the word to announce my affinity with a subculture that aspires to outlaw status. Each of these meanings enshrines some sort of little fib. As in the obvious fact that my outlaw status is belied by my helplessness, which causes any swaggering to possess a tinge of pathos. If I tried to swagger, I would fall down.

Because *cripple* is one of those somewhat archaic words that describes a population conventionally seen as oppressed, it now comes off as a slur when spoken in the company of upright citizens. We all know such words, slurs that are mainly racial and that take on a showboat quality when they come from the mouths of their intended targets. Even the word *nigger*, which has been called "the nuclear bomb of racial epithets," has had some air added to its final syllable and, in that inflated pronunciation, was turned into a shield by black comics and rap singers of the late twentieth century—they held up the shield and stood behind it. Would it have been more courageous for them to have stood without the shield? Now when it crops up in the news, in some recapitulation of its deliverance, it gets coded as *the N-word*, as a way of clarifying intention, of saying *I am not a racist* even though the expression *the N-word* is cloying, pathetic.

Perhaps it is the weak who take most pleasure in damning themselves, a sophomoric way of plumping up the pillow of the ego. While I was a cowering child I fell in love with the words *wop*, *dago*, and *guinea*, because Italians were the gladiators of my town, where we were not an insignificant minority—the vowels in our last names clanked like armor. I was not tough, only half a dago, but thought some metal might flake off the words and adhere to me. And so I rehearsed them with abandon. When I mentioned this the other day to a man who was born in Italy, he looked at me with horror and pity as he poured a drop of anisette into his espresso's tiny cup.

Dago from the Spanish for James, *Diego*—somehow the nationalities got swapped around. The derivation of *wop* is more murky: it could mean *dandy*, or could mean *sour wine*. *Guinea* from *Guinea Negro*, a linkage between Africans and people from southern Italy, forged by the dark skin I don't possess. This was the name we loved best, the one that alluded to the coveted brown tint—the darker the skin, the more status attached, dark people being exotic, rare, associated with danger. *Guinea!* we yelled as we pushed each other off the floating dock and into the toxic river, in which we guineas were not afraid to swim, though I sometimes wonder if those poisoned waters were what damaged my immune system, causing it to attack my brain.

To me it seems illogical that a word should be permitted to some people and not to others. The problem is intention, I suppose, the assumption being that a member of a community can use an old (corroded by time, or cruel history, to now become appalling) label in a manner that expresses brotherhood while at the same time armoring the community against those who would besiege it. The intentions of outsiders, on the other hand, can't be so easily trusted. This assumes that the distinction between insider and outsider is easy to make: we need to know skin tone or the number of vowels in a name. The urban accent or the wheelchair. To get permission to say *cripple*, I have to let people see me. And I don't like people to see me. This is the beauty of words, how they allow speech without having to be seen. So *cripple* leads to a conundrum: I have to be seen/I don't want to be seen.

The word also has an antique feel, like a butter churn, like some remnant of the vocabulary of grandparents from the Old World. To make the label more aggressive, and maybe chummier, the brotherhood of those foiled by bad body-luck sometimes shortens it to *crip*, as in: *the crip community*. Never having been much of a club-joiner, however, I find myself too aloof for the bonhomie of *crip*.

My friend Marva, whose family calls her *gimp*, says that this name did sting at first, though she assumes they use it to assure her she's not being pitied. When she asked what I am called, I realized that my family doesn't call me anything. They do not refer to *my condition*, not wishing to appear ill-bred. Earlier in my disease they were probably as stunned and stymied as I was—and in those days it seemed possible to evade the body if we simply did not speak of it. This was a proven tactic, which had served us well in regard to sex.

Now, when backed into a corner, my family calls me *disabled*, the static electricity clumping into quotation marks around the word. *Disabled* isn't cloying exactly, though it does strike me as overly sanitized in its depiction of a state that is so oftentimes a mess.

My dislike for *disabled* comes from its being cobbled together from negation: *not* able, like *in*-valid. I cling to the fantasy that I could do anything with the right technology, which only the economies of scale have worked against—by now there ought to be some kind of robotic superstructure to stand me up and walk me. Or a lightweight jetpack (because as early as the mid-1960s Bell Aerosystems had invented barrels and chairs that flew, all this technology prior to the electronic age that shrunk the phone booth into something smaller than a cigarette pack). One can only assume that the fear of litigation halted the development of jetpacks or electric bones that would let the cripples march.

There it is again, the word. *In your face* we say of people who like to invade social boundaries. All my life I have had trouble with being able to correctly gauge the boundary's circumference—I think I suffer from a mild form of dyslexia that has waltzed me through a life of blunders. *Describe me,* I asked my friend Vivian, who also calls herself a cripple. She taught art at the Wa He Lut Indian School, where a girl born with fetal alcohol syndrome once asked fearfully: *What's wrong with you?*

When Vivian asked what she meant, the girl said: *I mean how you're crimpled.*

Vivian tells me: *You'll blurt out anything that pops into your head,* and I think that my tendency to blurt comes from my being such a blank slate, the suburban girl with barely any history. A good student, but not too good. Not bad enough to be interesting in a James Dean sort of way, just a likeable whiner, a slacker before the coinage of the word. On the high school track team, I often stopped to walk.

And now at last I do have a unique identity, though it is not at all what I envisioned—still better than nothing, I sometimes think. Now I am: *bag lady on a cart jury-rigged with lights and crutches.* Know me slightly, and I am disarmed sufficiently to qualify as a *kook*. Know me well, and I become merely an *eccentric*.

The name I find most accurate to my current state is a word our society has circled half a rotation past: *handicapped*, derived from the eighteenth-century manner of wagering by placing money in a cap. Perhaps America abandoned the word because of the folksiness of its constituent parts, the words *handy* and *cap*, which seem too slight for the body's grueling saga. But my affection for the word comes from one of my primal reading experiences, a story by Kurt Vonnegut called "Harrison Bergeron" that was first published in 1961, when I was three. I must have read it in junior high, and now, looking at it for the first time in over thirty years, I see that though its version of Big Brother futurism is hammered out with a heavy mallet, the central image still appeals to me.

In the story a married couple is watching a ballet on TV, the dancers weighted with "sash-weights and bags of birdshot, and their faces were masked, so that no one, seeing a free and graceful gesture or a pretty face, would feel like something the cat drug in." Those who are smart (like the husband) must wear earphones through which the government broadcasts loud noises so they can't think.

To be weighted with canvas sacks full of pellets turns out to be a not-bad approximation of what my body actually *feels* like (sacks of pellets and nettles). The bags are tied to my ankles so I can't lift my legs, and it spooks me that in junior high school I would have so deliberately filed the story in my brain's otherwise jumbled cabinet, that the body would broadcast its secret future so brazenly.

There is also a genteel quaintness associated with *handi-capped*, versus the technological *disabled*. *Crippled*, on the other hand, comes out of the gnomic European setting of fairy tales, which is the basis of its appeal. The plot may be topsy-turvy, but we trust that it will be untwisted at the end. The plot may be cruel and gruesome, but it is often hopeful nonetheless.

My small city shares some qualities with the weird nocturnal settings of fairy tales, in that its streets are clogged with young people at night, the primary colors of their hair massaged into phantasmagoric shapes. Sometimes I'll be rolling along the streets and a shout will ring from the dampness and the dark—*Cripple!* This will unhinge me not because the word is offensive but because I realize how visible I am, how I have lost, forever and utterly, the ability to blend in. All my life, isn't this what I aspired toward—being a distinctive someone? And haven't I, like the protagonist of the fairy tale, finally gotten what was once my fervent wish?

Medicine

1

First thing that happened, after I got diagnosed with the disease, was that my mother urged me to see the famous holistic doctor in Seattle. I was surprised to find his office in a strip mall, his waiting room under perpetual construction, with sheets of milky plastic flapping across holes where doors and windows had once been. This gave an especially pathetic aspect to the stricken, who looked like citizens of a Soviet republic that no longer existed. Perhaps because they trembled in their winter coats.

Oh right, I had to remind myself, *now you are one of the stricken.*

Perhaps because we trembled in our winter coats.

2

The famous holistic doctor could not retain in his care all those who made appeals, so he passed me along to another doctor in his clinic, a woman whose pink complexion I took to be an indicator of health. But she was very fat, and this made me suspicious of her advice, which pertained mainly to my diet and my ingestion of the expensive vitamins she had me buy (which were sold by the doctor's office). Simultaneously, I felt queasy about my prejudice regarding her size, which revealed the shallowness of my character. So I returned diligently to my appointments although she also had an irksome habit of hugging me before I left.

For a while I carried around a knapsack full of vitamin bottles. In those days my sorrow eased up rarely, and whenever it did I felt like a drenched person who suddenly finds herself standing in a sunbeam shooting through a gap in the thunderheads.

Because I was both young and sad, during this phase of my treatment I also went to London to track down a man I loved, and there the slaking happened when I found an exhibit in the British Museum of watercolors by the poet William Blake. They were displayed behind little velvet curtains so as not to be faded by even the dim museum light. Each time I lifted my arm to lift the cloth, the vitamins rattled like an aboriginal percussion instrument, a gourd full of soft pebbles, background music that played while I peeked at Nebuchadnezzar crawling on his knees and Satan inflicting the boils on Job, a painting that spooked me with its eerie familiarity until I realized that I'd had the poster in my college dorm room.

3

The doctor in practice with the famous holistic doctor urged me to remove the fillings in my teeth because they contained the toxin mercury. She recommended a dentist in Tacoma who specialized in this procedure. The filling particles were so poisonous that his assistant used a device like a Dust-buster to suck them away as he worked with his drill.

The dentist instructed me to drink a special soup called "Bieler's Broth," which contained a variety of green vegeta-bles cooked in bouillon. I felt foolish making it from his recipe, particularly when it came time to drink. Its banal taste insulted me for some inexplicable reason.

Yet what I liked about this guy was how he didn't engage in the annoying trademark behavior of dentists: asking ques-tions when one's mouth is full of tools. Instead he kept up a steady comic patter with his Dustbustering assistant, while his office stereo played what is sometimes known as "novelty music." In particular I remember the song "Guitarzan," a semi—spoken-word number that gave both the dentist and his assistant the chance to chime in, respectively, as Tarzan and Jane. Tarzan mumbled a low-pitched rhyme, while Jane's high wail was supposed to conjure a woman clinging to a vine, swooping through the trees.

4

My co-workers at the small college where I worked of course gave me advice about alternative forms of healing that they'd found to be of use. An education professor gave me a book by the famous Ayurvedic doctor who'd not yet become famous. In the book he made an obvious point that nonetheless was stunning to me: how the mind says *Now my leg will move* and a complex biochemical process is unleashed that in fact causes the leg to move.

So I thought: *Now my leg will move.* But it didn't.

5

And a sociology professor gave me the name of her Chinese doctor in Seattle. His office was in the international district, near the pet store I loved whose narrow aisles were crowded with fish tanks. The tanks invariably contained dead fish, which nobody got exercised enough about to remove. I read this as a sign of clearheadedness—mortality was not to be feared. I think that's why I loved the store, despite the way it stank.

The doctor's English was barely decipherable to me, and I understood that I represented just a small subset of his patients too stupid to be able to speak Chinese. He responded the same way Americans do when traveling abroad and wishing to be understood—he made his voice so loud I cowered.

Stick out your tongue! he commanded. Then he consulted his big book of tongues, whose photos' lurid colors so contrasted with their orderly array that they left me dizzy.

It is the liver! he shouted after a few minutes of flipping. Taking a Q-tip and unwinding the cotton from one of its ends, he stabbed a spot inside my ear. I understood him when he said I should do this throughout the day, I should stab hard enough to hurt.

6

When I first moved to this town, there was only one thera-pist who practiced the technique called Jin Shin Jitsu. She also was a counselor, so our sessions comprised two distinct halves. First I would weep and then she would touch me.

She placed her hands on two different topographical fea-tures of my body—say, nose and shoulder—creating a kind of circuit while soothing music played. Soothing music an-noys me until my annoyance builds up enough momentum to burst through to surrender like the car leaping through the paper skin inside the hoop of flame. Then I can stand the soothing music.

But I grew suspicious, as our weeks of weep-and-touch went by, that she wanted to cut down on the weeping and up the touching half. I got the impression she didn't think I was gaining ground on my misery quickly enough. And was it just me, or had she changed her manner of offering the tis-sue box? Where once had been her tentative nudge, now there was a disgruntled thrust?

7

It was in my hunt to score some vitamin B shots that I learned of Dr. N, whose office I found—oddly—in a residential apartment complex south of town. The person who mentioned his name was the same woman who'd sent me to the Chinese doctor in Seattle, and she confided that, though she knew he gave the shots, she wouldn't necessarily recommend him. She'd seen him for a case of strep throat and had allowed him to give her a pelvic exam because he said he needed to check for signs of yeast. Then she learned other women had filed complaints. Though her humiliation obviously pained her, she said she was grateful for his recipe for a delicious soup that she still made.

No, she said in answer to my question, it was not called Bieler's Broth.

Dr. N himself answered the door of his apartment/office, which was long and narrow, with a windowless storage room between the front office (no receptionist) and the back bedroom, which served now as his examination room. Before he gave me the shot, he asked a dozen standard questions. When he asked if I had any sexual dysfunction, I asked him why he wanted to know, though I am usually not assertive in the presence of authority.

"Sexual dysfunction is indicative of many underlying conditions," he answered, backpedaling but not quite defensive: it seemed as if he knew I knew. But soon he gave up on his line of questioning and administered the shot into my buttocks, after I cinched down my skirt as few inches as necessary in the storage room.

Afterward he said, "I believe there is hope for you. I had another patient with multiple sclerosis who came here cry-

ing"—here he did a pantomime of a woman in distress—
"and now she is getting married, after I made her better."

He lifted his shirt and swatted his chest with the back sides
of his hands. "Guess how old I am!" *Fifty?* "Almost sixty!
And I win swimming competitions with men half my age."

And his body *was* remarkably taut—it was only his eyes
that looked defeated, their black interiors like prunes—or
some other kind of shriveled, desiccated fruit.

8

Soon I learned that I could get the vitamin shots from a
naturopath. The one whose office was nearest where I
worked specialized in colon irrigation. She wore heels and
tight-fitting, brightly colored business suits that did not
flatter her figure.

This amused me because, soon into our first meeting, she
told me about how she'd been so constipated as a child that
she moved her bowels only once a week. Her parents kept a
stick by the toilet so she could chop her stools before she
flushed. Though she must have told the story all the time, it
amused her too, so much so that afterward she'd used a tis-
sue to blot the mascara stains that were ruining the rest of
her make-up, before she signaled that it was time to return to
more sober work by hitching down her skirt where it had
ridden up her thighs, having skidded along the shimmering
surface of her nylons.

9

Kombucha is the name of a rubbery fungus that resembles a moon-glo frisbee. My first job associated with its care was to procure a large pickle jar to keep it in, as though it were a pet like a snake in need of a terrarium.

It lived by floating—quivering it seemed—on a lagoon of sweet green tea. Clouds and specks and ghostly tentacles appeared, drifting below it in the jar. Fermentation caused the tea to taste like apple cider vinegar, and each day I was supposed to siphon off a cup to drink. The brew was said to have healing powers that I never investigated too thoroughly, though my mushroom, which I obtained from a friend, came with a sheaf of Xeroxed testimonials.

Kombucha replicates by spawning a twin, a flat clone that grows slowly until its thickness equals the parent's. This meant that each week brought a new fungus to be given away, and soon all my friends had their own mushrooms—the mushroom's curative powers were general enough to suit all our needs. Our collective fungal propagation came to be a civic rite that required an ever-increasing group of participants, like a pyramid or Ponzi scheme, and everybody knew it couldn't go on forever.

The end may have been foreshadowed in all the ghost-gook our creatures produced. We didn't stare at our jars too long. Soon we began procrastinating about the chores of making their tea and pulling apart the new offspring, until we all had layer on layer of the tan mushrooms, pleated like accordions left to rot in tannic puddles in the middle of a rainy woods.

10

The friend who gave me the mushroom that united so many of us for just a season lived on a shoestring, yet she invested in an expensive machine called *The Voyager*. When I asked her recently how she came to possess it, she didn't remember: the afflicted are never at a loss for people who show up on their doorstep with a tool or a pill to sell. This is a form of celebrity, to learn that one's name is being whispered in far-off rooms. And yet the vendors seem sincere when they arrive at the door with their products, which they look down at so hopefully, as if they held a new baby in their arms.

The Voyager could be set to various modes: *Relaxation, Energy, Sleep*. Put on its black visor and shooting stripes or dots appeared, like when you hurt yourself and reflexively your eyes clamp shut.

When my friend loaned me The Voyager, I found its pain-lessness disorienting: its visions looked like they'd been birthed by trauma and so I thought pain should accompany them. Every so often I'd take The Voyager off to orient myself once again to the non-Voyager world. Then I'd scan myself and become angry when nothing hurt.

11

Evening primrose oil, niacin, olive extract, garlic, flaxseed oil, grape seed extract, [forgotten herb X], ginseng, bioflavinoids, [forgotten supplement Z], lecithin, Coenzyme Q_{10}. Though I forget why I took them, some names I remember simply for their jangly quilt of syllables: Pycnogenol, Sphingolin. This last pill was made from cow brains, and I thought it made sense to ingest the neural coating that my immune system was attacking. If I ate a bit each day, I thought my body might get used to it. Then mad cow disease made my theory seem imprudent.

Often the vitamin salesperson was someone I knew vaguely, like the man who was supposed to install carpet in my home. I'd buy the pills for a while, and the clinking of my coins became the music to which I danced with these peddlers before they ebbed away.

12

The strange thing about the Bee Lady was that she charged a pittance for her services. She lived in a fine home by the water, distinguished by the lovely gardens she'd created on its grounds. Her bee work occurred in a rustic cabin amid the vegetables and flowers. My friend had been getting stung three times a week, building up her tolerance. Now that the stings belong to the middle ground of her past, she says they ruined her life: "puking, burning, in pain . . . etc." But all I could think of was Peter Rabbit when I went with her to the Cabin of Stings.

The Bee Lady had pulled sixty bees from their hive before we came. She kept them in a jar where she sprayed them with honey solution to keep them calmly engaged in their compulsive grooming. My friend lay facedown shirtless on a table while the bee lady extracted them one at a time with a pair of wooden tongs. By pressing bee to skin, she coaxed it to sting, making two broad stripes that ran down both sides of my friend's spine. After each bee had stung she put it into a different jar, the jar of goners.

She left all the stingers in place until the end. They looked like tiny black rose thorns when finally she tweezed them out.

Then she asked if I wanted to be stung—this seemed a too-conscious act of charity, and reflexively I refused it. But I was glad she coaxed me until I pointed shyly to my knee. One more bee in the dead jar, and I too was admitted into the club of pain.

13

Though I was skeptical by now, hope niggled me, as always, when I entered the famous psychic healer's house. Because it was the students of the psychic healer and not the psychic healer herself who'd be doing the healing, it was being of-fered free. This made me wonder if the healing would be second-rate.

My hope percolated partly from the fact that I'd walked with my crutches through her muddy yard. I even climbed unaided into my designated elevated cot, though in my en-thusiasm I forgot to take off my shoes. When this was called to my attention I removed them before settling back into place while the psychic healer gave her introductory speech. She announced that she was going to name her school after the wizard school in the Harry Potter books.

There were many cots set up in her living room: one student each. With the shades drawn against the day, the air full of motes, she said the students were going to form a net of energy. We could expect sensations of such profundity that they might cause us to weep, and afterward we might even see "manifestations"—particles of matter on our cots where our illness had fallen out of our bodies.

Then the dulcimer music began to ding, and the students made the net. I squinted and thought I could even see the rays of energy between them. Time collapsed like a telescope: I think I fell asleep. When the lights came up, we were all given cups of water.

My student said: "Look, you have manifestations."

A few brown specks like mouse turds lay on the sheet. For a moment I grew elated to see how my disease had fallen out.

Then I remembered the mud on my shoes.

"No, I think these are manifestations," my student said. And the psychic healer was called over for consultation. Manifestations, yes!

The room erupted then, all because of me.

14

The pale homeopath had sad, limp hair. Her office was only open part-time because she had to take dialysis every other afternoon.

She gave me a physical exam and questioned me in detail about my youth. "What about my youth?" I said, and she said, you know, what kind of kid I was. I described myself as moody, and when she asked me to elaborate I said, for example, I remember daydreaming more than once about taking a kitchen knife and stabbing it into my chest. All my answers she recorded in detailed notes.

Then she looked up my condition in the big musty ancient homeopathy book that a man she called her mentor had written. Every morning he poured a pitcher of ice water down his spine, and she urged me to do the same. And she gave me the tiniest of yellow pills that, under scientific scrutiny, would be found to contain only sugar—this she freely admitted.

One part active substance, diluted a millionfold.

She concluded by reading back the notes she'd taken to make sure she had recorded all pertinent information: *you day-dreamt of stabbing a kitchen knife into your chest*, and she said this quickly and without emotion, as if it were a summary of the weather.

15

The other day I saw my former acupuncturist at the farmers' market. He's hard to recognize because he is short now, whereas he was once a tall man with a wild fringe of dark hair that circled his head like a lion's mane and which lent a devilish, or maybe I should say wizardly, aspect to his appearance. He looked as if he should have been wearing a robe covered in stars. But he wore sweatpants to indulge his catlike movements.

What caused his growing shorter was the disintegration

of his spine, from a form of bone cancer that should have killed him but didn't. His shrinkage does not seem as much of a transformation as his rigid posture does. No more cat.

When I ask how he accounts for his survival, he tells me he did both Eastern medicine and Western, alternative and mainstream; he flew to Europe, he tracked down every remedy and tried them all. I know that for a while we both walked with crutches, but then he got better while I got worse. Our conversation flags when it becomes obvious that our luck is riding opposite seats on fortune's wheel.

But I don't want to be so miserly of spirit as to be jealous. Instead I salute him: *Soldier carry on!* Then stiffly he ambles off, down the aisles of organic vegetable stalls, which have been erected under white tents like the field hospitals of the Civil War.

16

Stabilized Aloe Vera Gel, Emu Oil (7%), Methylsulfonyl Methane, Oleyl Alcohol (and) Zanthoxylum Alatum Extract, Horse Chestnut Extract, Comfrey Extract, Calendula Extract, Chamomile Extract, Vitamins A, D3, and E, Glucosamine Sulfate, Allantoin, Panthenol, Diazolidinyl Urea.

This is a list of the active ingredients in the superstrength Blue Emu cream I've just bought. For three days now I have been using it to see if it will ease the burning in my lower legs. So far the doctors have not been able to come up with anything that soothes the pain, nor have acupuncture needles helped. But since this emu cream . . . hard to tell. It costs twelve dollars for a two-week supply, which my mainstream doctor considers a rip-off. He may not know that its main ingredient comes from a gland in the anus of that giant vicious bird.

Job versus Prometheus

Might as well start with my legs, which feel like . . . what? Giraffes whose necks are bandaged with sandpaper? Burning trees being evacuated by squirrels with sharp claws? Fence-posts sunk into two holes full of concrete? Concrete that's been wetted down with acid? These descriptions are somewhat accurate, but at the same time they seem too cute. At the pain clinic where I go to have the computer pump that's implanted in my body refilled with muscle relaxants, when the doctor (whom I call Doctor Dreamboat) asked me if my pain felt like pins and needles, I said: "No, it's more like rubbing against a hot driveway impregnated with broken glass—" and Doctor Dreamboat cut me off with one of those doctorly semi-chuckles and said, "Oh right, you're the poet."

Montaigne called pain the "worst accident of our being" (*the very trees seem to groan at the blows that are given them*), and yet any description comes off as self-indulgent because to speak of pain is considered to be in bad taste. Nobody likes a whiner. Forget the old women whose mustaches quiver. That's why people took refuge in this country—to get away from those who felt no compunction about such extreme displays as slapping themselves and wailing with grief. Pain does not make for good conversation because the purpose of conversation is to elicit more conversation, and if you tell someone you want to chop off your legs the talk will come to a halt (Jim made the mistake of telling a co-worker about the leg-chopping, and she asked, wincing, if I knew about the phenomenon called *phantom pain*).

As for Jim, whenever I ask him to fetch the ax he says it makes him think of his grandmother, about whom he remembers little but that she lived on toast and boiled potatoes, fed him chicken-loaf sandwiches, and wore shoes that had room for her big toes to air their bunions. Whenever I wake up with my leg-chopping complaints, he starts to wail the mantra she recited: *Oh the pain, Jimke! Oh the pain, the pain!*

.   .   .   .   .

The poet Louise Glück traces the impulse to talk about subjects that are supposed to be forbidden back to Eve and her apple:

> In the myth of the Garden, the forbidden exerts over the susceptible human mind irresistible allure. The force of this allure is absolute, final; the fact of it shapes, ever afterward, human character and the human vision of human destiny. The myth's potency derives from the fact that there is no going back: exile and contamination occur once, the explicit descent which is the lovers' punishment becomes a permanent burden or affliction. Which is to say: the myth is tragic.

Glück insists that tragedy means there is no going back, no rising above fate, and to tack onto tragedy some kind of ending that implies redemption falsifies the story—or at least rejects the story's mythic dimension.

As a kid, I found original sin a particularly terrifying myth to be burdened with—though I admit to being turned on by the fact that Adam and Eve were naked. Their suffering left me puzzled, though: okay, they had to leave the Garden for a life spent wandering around dressed in leaves. Was that so bad? The way important details were left out drove me nuts. Like what the weather was like outside the Garden—was it cold, or did they lead the free-and-easy life of the muddy nudists at Woodstock?

Of course, the Old Testament's most famous sufferer is Job—a righteous man subjected to a series of tests that result from a sinister collaboration between God and Satan. First his livestock die, then his house falls down, killing his ten children. That final tragedy whizzes by in just a few words, though, with God delivering a case of boils to Job for the coup de grâce. The tragic story fizzles, and the poem becomes a debate between Job and three friends who try to tell him why he shouldn't wish for his own death. They don't make much headway until at last God himself shows up in a whirlwind to tell Job to knock it off with the pity-party.

And Job caves in, first by going silent: "I put my hand on my mouth. / I have said too much already; / now I will speak no more." Then God storms around some more from within his whirlwind, decorating his rant with beasts like the

Leviathan, like cheesy special effects at the climax of a movie. When, at the end, Job is completely debased, he reiterates his willingness to hold his tongue: "Therefore I will be quiet, / comforted that I am dust." (This translation, by Stephen Mitchell, softens the self-loathing of the King James Version, which goes: *I abhor myself and repent in dust and ashes.*)

Once Job agrees to quit whining, God gives him his wealth back, along with ten more children of the exact same gender-ratio as the first set, and these new children even seem to be an improvement on the original ones, judging by the fact that this time around we learn their names, at least the beautiful daughters' names—Dove, Cinnamon, and Eye-Shadow, in Mitchell's translation. The dead children disappear without a trace, and no one seems too broken up about it.

.   .   .   .   .

The other day I tuned in to a documentary about the children who live in the area surrounding the Chernobyl nuclear plant, many of whom have grotesque birth defects. They were difficult to look at, and my first impulse was to flee by channel-surfing away, but I caught myself and said: *What a poseur—you want to write about tragedy and you can't even bring yourself to look.* So I stuck it out with those kids, those whose heads were shaped like Bartlett pears and those whose brains grew in sacs outside their skulls. I would have liked to hear them speak about their lives, but they were not capable of speech—their experience would remain off-limits to me. I could not enter their lives or bodies and *look out from* within them.

Sometimes I imagine I'm the one on TV and my friends are watching. (*Do they think my life is tragic?*) This mental exercise will only lead to trouble. Better to stay inside the dwindling brain than to indulge in the thought-experiment of entering another brain and taking a glance at the self, although it might be more socially acceptable for someone else to write about me than for me to write about myself, as I'm doing here, what with the good taste/unspeakability problem that arises when a life marked by what are seen conventionally as tragic parameters (pain, debility, blah-blah, death) is described from within.

You might argue: *Whoa, don't try to tell me I haven't seen people blabbering about their body-troubles* . . . say on the kind of TV talk shows *where the sufferer might win a car!* But of course this is spectacle, the outside view. Also, on this talk-TV where people bare themselves, the only story that's permissible is the one that ends with upward motion and not the slipping down. You can't tell your story if it does not rise; good taste demands that the person who is stuck inside disease withdraw from public view.

We do have a few accounts—Willem de Kooning's last paintings, made during his prolific dementia. Or Jean-Dominique Bauby's memoir, *The Diving Bell and the Butterfly*, written after a stroke left him with "locked-in syndrome"— he dictated the book by blinking his left eye. Or there's even this report from Emerson's old age: "I have lost my mental faculties but am perfectly well."

.   .   .   .   .

Our longstanding authority on the subject of tragedy is Aristotle, who wrote about the subject in his *Poetics*. What tragedy does to its audience, he says, is arouse *pity and fear*, so that the audience gets to experience these emotions in a contained sort of setting—presumably as an alternative to experiencing them as they normally do, in life itself. People went to the ancient plays with their downward-skidding plots in order to purge their minds of imagining that this sort of future lay in waiting for themselves.

Aristotle does not talk about what happened when the audience went home and still found maybe Pa, maybe Junior, dying in a back room, as must have often been the case. Art can perform the service of catharsis, but it can't cure a body or whisk it away, and the best the play could hope to do was to leave people better steeled for the loved one's demise. There in the theater, though, a person is allowed to do the un-useful thing and fall apart, and other people in the audience are sure to be weeping too. So no one needs to feel absurd about losing his or her mind for a little while.

(In the early days of my disease, I suspected my friends of presenting a false front if they weren't willing to go a little crazy with me. I wanted us to get crazed and drunk and beat our breasts and rip our tunics and rage and weep, which is what the ancient poets tell us to do if we are to respond to bad news in authentic manner. But lately I'm less inclined to that kind of falling-apart. When faced with a crisis like grief over the fallen house, the kind of person you want hanging around is someone who is handy with a hammer, somebody like the manic-whirlwind energetic God who knows how to get the house rebuilt.)

One essential aspect to a successful tragic plot, according to Aristotle—and this is art I'm talking about, I need to maintain the distinction between tragedy in art and tragedy in life, a distinction oddly smudged in many scholarly discussions of the subject—is that it should be quick, or quickish: the action "endeavors to keep as far as possible within a single circuit of the sun, or something near that." It also should be complete in itself, a whole that has a beginning, middle, and end. "Beauty is a matter of size and order, and therefore impossible either (1) in a very minute creature, since our perception becomes indistinct as it approaches instantaneity, or (2) in a creature of vast size—one, say, a thousand miles long—as in that case, instead of the object being seen all at once, the unity and wholeness of it is lost to the beholder."

This is where art and life part company. Thanks to high-tech surgical excisions and pharmaceutical assaults on the body, the form that tragedy now takes in life is often a slowish downward slide, which doesn't suit the demands of literature because it is too big and long. (Thomas Hardy found this out when he wrote his novel *Jude the Obscure*—with its long, relentlessly plunging trajectory—and was savaged by critics, to the point that the book was burned. He then turned to writing lyric poems, their brevity giving him the freedom to air his laments.)

．　．　．　．　．

I have plenty of friends who will not watch movies if their plotlines plunge. As a culture we have little use for lamentation and instead choose laughter for our cathartic agent. So why, then, does tragedy make up the bulk of the stories that we lug with us into the future? We remember Macbeth and Hamlet and King Lear better than we remember all of Shakespeare's happy lovers. The tormented are more indelible.

"It is not the worst," says a character in *Lear*, "so long as we can say it is the worst." This sounds reasonable enough until you remember *oh Jimke the pain the pain* and the unspeakable desire to chop off the legs. Shakespeare hadn't reckoned on modern medicine's ability to attenuate disease, nor had his almost-contemporary Michel de Montaigne, who dispensed with the problem of pain by stating that if it was intense, it would be over soon, or, if it wasn't intense, it could be withstood. Pain that was intense and long could be found in only the goriest myths. If you want to hear about that kind of pain, your man is Prometheus.

．　．　．　．　．

Though I never studied Greek or Latin, I do have on my shelf a small collection of ancient tragedies. Other people must have been eager to be rid of them, seeing as these books came from the kind of used-book sales where, if you arrive at their tail ends, you are charged by the number of brown paper shopping bags you fill. These were the books that no-body wanted to read, or could bear to read, and I bought them in my youth because I was eager to smarten myself up, though I could not pronounce the name Aeschylus.

I knew who Prometheus was, though—the god who got chained in a crag so his liver could be pecked out by eagles. The story is a profound one for anyone who lives in the grip of a nonlethal illness, as his liver mysteriously regenerates each night so the attack can be repeated—"each changing hour will bring successive pain / to rack / your body"—and since he is immortal, he can't just die and escape his pains.

Zeus has ordered this perpetual torment because Prometheus stole fire from the other gods and gave it to men. But that was not his worst offense, he who could see the future, his name meaning "wise before the event." He also made it possible that humans no longer foresaw their deaths. Instead, Prometheus had "planted firmly in their hearts blind hopefulness."

The worst thing about disease is how it undoes Prometheus's good deed and gives the patient a flash glimpse at his or her possible death—a flash that's never exactly accurate, of course, because we all ride the plotlines of our singular, inevitable physical demise. Disease is notoriously inconsistent. And yet the flash is still horrifying, frightening beyond belief, because it might contain some truth after all.

Aeschylus's *Prometheus Bound* describes the god's crucifixion, the result of his unwillingness to say he's sorry for his deeds. The poem about Prometheus is of the same approximate vintage as the poem about Job, though Prometheus is the anti-Job, steadfast in his refusal to give up lamenting his fate. Sarcastically, he tells his tormentors: "Oh, it is easy for the one who stands outside / The prison-wall of pain to exhort and teach the one / Who suffers." Unlike Job, who starts with this kind of sarcasm and is coaxed—then divinely commanded—away from it, Prometheus never gives it up.

The catharsis that's supposed to come from watching a tragic drama is the final revelation that its victim is not us after all. We walk out of the theater and discover that we are not pinioned on the rock; our children, in fact, are home with the babysitter. This is the problem tragic art presents to those who live at the center of tragedy, or at least what could be called tragedy from the outward view. The center-dwellers have too much in common with the protagonist.

But suffering is also transformed into something else when you're the one looking outward from inside of it—I shouldn't have even called it suffering. No one lives at the center of the tragedy because at the center there *is* no tragedy, the way a fish in a bowl doesn't see the bowl, instead it sees the distorted world beyond. From the outside, it may look like my body has become more still, but it's a stillness that's also busy. Busy with the complex logistics of getting from place A to B, and busy also with its inner life, the inner life that grows so large it consumes the body. In my case, I hope the sufferer has turned into a sentinel, trying to figure out which bird gave that shrill cry outside the window, the cry that sounded like it could have come from a red-tailed hawk.

And so with Prometheus, who keeps his eye on the landscape even while the eagles shred him:

Now it is happening: threat gives place to performance.
The earth rocks; thunder, echoing from the depth,
Roars in answer; fiery lightnings twist and flash.
Dust dances in a whirling fountain;
Blasts of the four winds skirmish together,
Set themselves in array for battle;
Sky and sea rage indistinguishably.
The cataclysm advances visibly upon me,
Sent by Zeus to make me afraid.

O Earth, my holy mother,
O sky, where sun and moon
Give light to all in turn,
You see how I am wronged!

Then the stage set falls down with a crash, and the people in the audience reenter the world of their own concerns, consoled because, no matter what their troubles, they've just seen someone whose fate is worse. Or consoled because they're now free to go home and wail, having just seen someone who's not afraid to keep lamenting, even when faced with an atmospheric showdown.

Job, on the other hand, shuts up at last when God unleashes the Leviathan and nature goes crazy. I like to think my own song oscillates between these two polarities of complaint: *Bitch bitch. Tweet tweet.*

Inside / Outside

A friend recently asked me: "Have you ever walked by a shop-window in a new hat you've just bought"—this was a man's hat he was talking about, probably purchased from the haberdashery downtown that's been in business thirty years despite the fact that I've never seen anyone go in or out, a shop patronized by ghosts only, ghosts plus my bald friend—"and you study yourself for a minute before you devilishly give the hat a tilt?"

"Oh no," was my answer, "I never stop to look. My advice would be *don't ever* stop to look."

For a while I taught remedial English at a college attached to a Benedictine monastery. Though I didn't understand how anyone could find happiness in monastic life (bad food, no sex), my religious colleagues inspired my envy for one reason: they could wear robes to work. Long black robes under which they wore jeans or old sweatpants or even their pajamas. In these garments they vanished the way the *Star Trek*

Enterprise became invisible once the technology called *the cloaking device* was engaged.

Out on the streets, where the robes had the opposite effect and made them ultra-visible, they opted for the camouflage of jeans and sweaters. The only sign of their being monks would be the expensive sandals they wore year-round.

In college I had a friend named Tom who wore a similar black robe that his sister sewed for him because he'd taken the notion that if he wore a garment that almost completely covered him he could almost completely disappear. One afternoon, when he went walking to the outskirts of our small Canadian village, a ring of children gathered around him, as if they'd been swept up from the twilight itself. And even though he was a tall, imposing man, they started chanting, "Weirdo! Weirdo!" until he got scared and had to run. Of course, the robe also made him ultra-visible, though I'm not sure that that wasn't what he'd intended. Young people generally don't want to blend in.

This was the 1970s, a decade when we quoted Henry David Thoreau: *Beware any enterprise that requires new clothes,* which we took for a warning about the superficiality of the world. After collage I intended to head off to my own private Walden Pond, some remote place where I'd wear flannel or go naked, depending on the season. In those days I thought the obsession with self-presentation was a retrograde stage in human evolution, soon to pass. I fully expected that, by my middle age, the loan officer at the bank might be wearing a pair of farmer overalls.

(But no—he can have an earring and a well-groomed ponytail, but the overalls do not qualify as an adequate garment, not even on the dress-down Fridays.)

Now I see two flaws to my youthful thinking: my rags were themselves a fashion trend. I spent hours embroidering the patches on my jeans, and the sophistication of this needlework established a hierarchy of cool among my friends. Before I knew it, punk came into style, ripped clothes still the uniform, though you could no longer claim to be naïve about there being no artifice in your making of the image you presented to the world. People started paying a lot of money for old jeans, a status item. I stopped wearing them because I still wanted to present myself as anti-status, anti-money.

Flaw two: even the duck has breeding plumage. So there must be genuine biological imperatives that drive us to present ourselves in an attractive light, however I chastise my friends for choosing the beauties on the computer dating website. (When it comes to computer dating, I get most of my information from my wheelchair salesman, an actor whose head is covered with attractive blond tresses and whose palsied arm I never noticed until he showed me how his fingers spasmed when he tried to grip his pen.

"I'd rather kill myself than go back to dating," I say.

He offers helpfully: "There are computer dating sites for people in wheelchairs."

"That's just it!" I say. "I'd kill myself if I had to date me.")

I've read somewhere that a famous philosopher—Wittgenstein maybe—considered the objective self/subjective self conundrum, the inside view versus the outside one, for a brief while before concluding that the dilemma was immature and unsolvable.

My distaste for *seeing* my objective self—for having to have an objective self at all—preceded illness, so it's not entirely a manifestation of my fear of becoming disabled. It first occurred back when I headed into my pubescence, when I took up the hems of my turquoise polyester culottes, and voilà: hot pants. I was feeling pretty good about myself for the brainstorm of this transformation, until a boy made fun of me as I walked the trail through the woods that led me home from school. Furthermore, he pointed out that my shoes were made of cardboard. This I'd never noticed; in fact, I was quite proud of my two-tone, blue-gray wingtips with the stacked heel. But the edge of a wing was curling back, and sure enough I saw it: cardboard.

The 1970s were a decade filled with calamities of self-presentation, as the dashing young Elvis collided into the fat old one in the karate suit. Prior to my adolescence, I knew only my subjective body, which knew the secret handholds in the bark of every local tree. The body that rode no-handed on the hand-me-down bicycle and did not see itself doing so: these memories occupy the slots in my brain that I associate most with happiness. By junior high, they were over. Right around the time when I began to menstruate, when I went off to YMCA camp for a month and sat bleeding on the shore of the lake for weeks. I gained an external idea of myself but lost confidence in my body as a dependable vehicle, whose purpose had nothing to do with reproduction but only transport from place to place.

This was what made me start hiking alone, in the suburban woodlots at first, where I could be all body, all subject—something not seen. A decade later I began to love walking into the vast landscapes of the West, where you can almost hear the whooshing as the land gets large, and the body dwindles to a matchstick that becomes your one survival tool.

In his backyard in Camden, New Jersey, a place he transformed into a wilderness that he called Timber Creek, Walt Whitman wrote: "There come moods when these clothes of ours are not only irksome to wear, but are themselves indecent." He was only in his late fifties, yet he'd become partially paralyzed, in spite of his cunningly orchestrated public persona as the vigorous avatar of America in its entirety. To reclaim this former self, he created a ritual in this, his old-ish age: first he stripped and covered himself in mud, then he rinsed his body and scrubbed it pink before rinsing it again. Then he performed what he called "vocalism" by singing and reciting poems before long bouts of wrestling naked with the trees. This rejuvenation through nature worked, sort of; at least it gave him enough oomph to stagger through a few more years as the bard of the New World.

It's a common equation for poets to make, from nudity to purity. Billy Collins lampooned this belief in a poem that recounts the rituals one of his narrators goes through before sitting down to write. First the tea is made and then the clothes come off, and then:

> . . . I remove my flesh and hang it over a chair.
> I slide it off my bones like a silken garment.
> I do this so that what I write will be pure,
> completely rinsed of the carnal,
> uncontaminated by the preoccupations of the body.

This is a run-up to the climactic gag of the poem ("I should mention that sometimes I leave my penis on"), but it also contains a serious possibility that troubles me, how the body will contaminate whatever it's making if allowed to pester the writer with its pings and squawks.

In fact, I have become something of a nudist these days—at least a nude-ish nudist. Since my shins sizzle at the rasp of even the lightest silk, they go naked in all seasons. On my feet I wear boots made of sheep-fur because socks have come to feel like thorns. Through winter sleet I wear these boots, and shorts, cutting a figure unlike anyone I know except a schizophrenic woman who calls herself "the ghost of Jim Morrison." She too goes bare-legged, though she also favors headbands and ponchos that dip to a triangle below her waist. She looked strange until a few years ago, when a tidal wave of ponchos rode back into style.

In addition to my two "good" pairs of shorts, one of which, the khaki pair, I just realized the other day was badly stained, I have a collection of others that my husband has passed down to me when they became too threadbare for him to be willing to wear. I also have a few flannel shirts that belonged to my dead father, and though they too are now unraveling I can't bear to throw them out. I have some "normal" shirts of my own, but because I push myself in a wheelchair their sleeves are frayed at the wrist. And because I sit almost all my waking hours, some flab often pushes its way to light above the waistband of my shorts.

My paranoia leaves me feeling that I appear abnormal, to my mind absurd—with this *look* that I have not wrought or sought. I suppose I could "work on" the image I present to the world, but this would require too much collusion with my objective self. That person is free to amble around in the world, whoever she is, but I will not traffic with her at all. No thank you, I'll stay here inside my head where the hearth is always lit.

For my job at the monastery, which I arrived at with only a Smokey the Bear hat and a box full of park ranger uniforms, I bought some dowdy conservative clothes in the Goodwill store to camouflage my true self, which I envisioned then as "Amazon slut-poet of the wilderness," a persona I concocted to compensate for my insecurities. To further complicate my self-presentation, sometimes my brain felt as though it had been struck by a mild bolt of lightning: a wave passed from my nape to my temple, and in its wake I was left with no idea what I had been thinking. A couple of times a day I had to think my way back into my life from scratch. A theater professor asked me if I wanted her to train me to overcome my stage fright when she saw me swoon at the first faculty meeting when I stood up to introduce myself.

In addition to remedial English, I also taught some Japanese students, whom I led on nature walks down the labyrinthine sentences of Charles Dickens. The students often seemed to be weighted with sorrow that they lugged around on my behalf, and I could not fathom what I'd done to cause them to adopt this body language in my presence. All I could think of was that, at the Christmas party, I volunteered to lead off the singing of "Rudolph the Red-nosed Reindeer" and dove into a key not to be found in either our Western tonal scale or their Eastern one and which caused their faces to redden, as if my clothes had gotten blown off by a tornado. I remembered an Asian proverb: *One breaking of wind takes away the learning of an entire semester.*

When the Japanese students arrived at the beginning of the semester, they were escorted by a gracious older man who had at great expense procured a heavy gilt-framed mirror, more enormous than a standard sheet of plywood. Etched into it were the words *You Mirror*—which confused me at first. I thought it meant the mirror was supposed to be its own autonomous being: *Hey you! Mirror!* But then I learned that the students were supposed to pause before it, in order to consider the image they were presenting to the world.

Naturally, the job required me to be open to the mysteries of foreign cultures, but still I had to restrain myself to not take a hammer to that mirror. It summarized the injustice of having an objective self that moves in an external world—if it exists, I am not so sure—the world that is a processing plant, grinding the meat of the *me* and churning out the sausage of the *you*. And even though my limp was barely visible back then, I scurried by the mirror, wishing I were a vampire who would vanish in its gaze.

Last year's therapist said: *our society wants to make disabled people invisible.* I said that being invisible would be all right with me.

Another memory from college: my tall friend Janis jumping wildly and whipping her arms overhead, after we walked into a smoky upstairs loft in Montreal that was packed with people dancing. Janis making a joke by winking at me as she shouted into the din: *Look at me! Hey, everybody, look at me!* Her joke was that our exuberance was fueled by our vanity, our desire to be *seen*, a problem Janis solved later that semester by starving herself into a skeleton that was barely visible when she turned sideways.

More recently, Susan Sontag has written, in connection with the pictures of the prisoners confined in Iraq's Abu Ghraib prison: "To live is to be photographed, to have a record of one's life, and therefore to go on with one's life oblivious, or claiming to be oblivious, of the camera's nonstop attentions. But to live is also to pose. To act in the community of actions recorded as images." I try to shed this burden of modernity, this requirement that we be photographed and suffer through additional replications of our bodies. The actual one I have to live with is quite enough. "There is the deep satisfaction of being photographed," Sontag writes, "to which one is now more inclined to respond not with a stiff, direct gaze (as in former times) but with glee." But not me—I remain as stern as a Victorian before the lens.

This is undoubtedly a manifestation of my childish wish

to undo reality, this not-wanting the photograph to weld my objective presence to the wheelchair. If I were to rob a bank, the witnesses would identify me by the chair, even if I were Frankenstein. My green skin and scars and bolts would be noted as secondary observations. What could override the image—a chartreuse muumuu? A large fur hat like a guard at Buckingham Palace? Even if I wore nothing at all my nakedness would be subsumed.

A scholar might call the wheelchair *A Transcendent Signifier*. The only thing I can think of to put in it, to strip its black-hole type gravitational power—the way it sucks everything into it—is to put a bomb in the seat. Or a baby. A bomb and a baby might work best.

Animals go naked, and the duck in extravagant plumage is the exception, because ordinarily they want to blend in, they want to travel camouflaged. This generality has not prevented the evolution of bright-red poisonous frogs whose color announces their lethal meat and the danger of their being consumed. Or the evolution of what is known as *dazzle camouflage*, like the zebra's stripes or the loon's op-art breast and neck, configurations that prevent predators from being able to tell exactly where the prey is, by turning the body into a blurry confusion, especially when it's in motion.

The elk herd that stands far off in the meadow by the Saint John's River looks to me, at first, like either dead shrubs or bales of hay. My binoculars are not powerful enough to do much good, until finally the shrubs begin to move. I also make out their pale haunches, rimmed in darker brown, I presume as an erotic costuming, the crotchless panty of the animal world. The summer has been dry and the grass is spare, so the elk forage in the dust for the pale withered blades.

There's only one trail, running atop the levee that separates the meadow from the river. It leads to an old hunting blind that's been restored as a viewing blind. We gradually become aware that the bird noises we've been hearing, the squeals and whistles, are actually coming from the elk. I'd heard the word *bugling* used to describe their calls, and so I pictured an assertive tooting, but these are shy wooing sounds that seem wrongly scaled to the size of the animal. The muffled cries sound like a kettle that has not yet come to boil.

The males make the sound—this time of year, they wear ornate interlacing horns. I count just five of them, as opposed to maybe thirty females. It seems that the size of the headgear determines the male's status in the herd. One male wears a great scaffold with six pointy tips on each of his antlers, and he struts as if he's king of all the rest, who are mostly occupied with snuffling in the grass.

That the big male has a strand of lichen wrapped around his horns like a green feather boa apparently doesn't seem to affect his standing in the herd, even though he looks completely ridiculous as he leads the others in the direction of the parking lot. Ridiculous to me, and also a lesson—that one can go through life quite successfully without considering one's objective image presented to the world. A mirror would only enrage the big buck now. He would see a rival there, another male with a rack as big as his, and he would probably charge ahead and smash the mirror, thereby solving the problem.

A Cripple in the Wilderness

I used to be a naturalist, but, in all honesty, what I liked more than the names and facts and maybe even the sights of nature was the opportunity that being a naturalist gave me to walk around in the woods. For a while I worked at Mount Rainier, and, in the early summer, I liked to go to a place called Summerland, where I skied on slopes that were not too crevasse-covered or steep. Finding my way was difficult with the trail obliterated by snow, and I was vain about my willingness to go alone, though I looked like a child.

In my late teens I had spent my summers as a naturalist along the Appalachian Trail where it veers near New York City. Young people were dispatched in teams of two of the same gender to live in primitive cabins—no toilet, and our outhouse was a quarter mile away—where we ran nature programs for children from the city. We bathed in the lake and swam in the nude—now I realize that living there with no telephone or radio was probably the most dangerous immersion in nature I ever had. During those summers, female hikers were raped along the Appalachian Trail and even killed. But I never had a hard time with anyone except a man who, as was the custom of those days, gave me a hallucinogenic drug and returned in the middle of the night to pee on my tent.

In my mind, I survived by becoming aloof: naturalist as bitch. But this is silly, to imagine I was not vulnerable. A bullet makes no distinction between bitch and sweetie-pie.

Becoming handicapped has meant becoming a little more congenial, in that my accessing wilderness now requires collaboration, as on this day when my friends and I are headed up to Mount Rainier. For Angus, this is an opportunity to put more break-in miles on the Harley-Davidson Dynaglide motorcycle that he just purchased down near Portland. I had navigated him home with my car because he wasn't yet supposed to take the bike over fifty miles per hour, nor was he supposed to drive for long at a constant speed, and this meant we had to use the back roads, where the pages of maps he had spent days printing off the computer and highlighting and annotating were useless. The hundred miles took us five hours. At one point we drove in circles, which we noticed only because we passed an old barn painted with "Dr. Wilson's Remedy for Weak Women" twice.

When Angus starts the motorcycle, it attracts the notice of Bob, the man who is painting my house. I feel guilty going off on an excursion while Bob works, which is another concession that becoming handicapped requires—I pay other people to do my work. Having always painted my own houses, this is a bitter pill. I'm not even driving the car loaded with my electric scooter; my friend Becky is.

"Nice bike," Bob says, though Angus can't hear him above the noise of his pipes.

"He just bought it!" I yell back. Angus is a chubby bald man closing in on sixty. I don't know why I feel compelled to give out information as the Harley warms. "His wife died! He has not ridden a motorcycle for thirty years!"

Many of us can be made bold by grief.

You can see what people call *The Mountain* on clear days from our town, the main roads laid out to give a dead-on view of it when you head east. Three peaks make up its crown, like a molar tooth. Now that I am crippled, rarely do I go there, even though some of the trails are paved in order to protect the alpine meadows. So theoretically I could ride up them, and this is our bittersweet mission of the day. When the snow melts, flowers bloom in such profusion that the colors make you swoon.

We missed the peak flower-blooming weeks while we arranged our trip. My psychic tendencies lean toward disappointment and lament. We have missed the flowers! Becky assures me there will still be plenty, being the kind of woman who can peer into any cup and spot the trace of moisture that still resides. We're leading Angus out of the desecrated Northwest that has been manufactured recently by countless big-box stores and cheap tract homes. You have to stay right in town, close to the water, or else go into the wilderness— because what's between them is a place of death, the towns of no town, the quickly manufactured present, which has no soul. I can't imagine our strip malls fifty years hence: they will be torn down within a decade, or else they will be dusty and decayed, abandoned structures where squatters will set up camp. The giant supermarkets will someday house our slums.

So we leave them, good riddance, and rise into the foothills, after crossing Mashell Prairie and Ohop Valley. It has not rained all summer, and yet the valley somehow is a green dip between hills, a velvety swale without any desecration. This is where you finally catch your breath, and no one stops here. It's a hands-off place, a place where the riders in their vehicles stay put, as if they know better than to blight this ceaseless stunning bright bright green.

Then we rise into the clear-cuts, a thoroughly blighted place, where the small firs grow as high as a tall man's head in stands that are unnaturally dense. The forest has been ravaged, and yet the forest is making itself again, in a mutant, hypertrophic way. Environmentalists see the ravagement and the mutation; industry people see the resilient growth, and the human life span is too short to know which view will win.

But soon we leave the clear-cuts behind, as the road zips by Alder Lake. This summer, due to the lack of rain, the lakebed is a flat expanse of mud, sliced by rivulets and divided into planes of different color, colonized by different algae. The lakebed should be littered with driftwood, giant stumps with gnarly, webby roots. But this has all been carted off. In a random act of art, someone has created a horse and a fish with the only wood that's left.

In wetter years, I used to kayak on this lake. The trip that gnaws most on my memory is one on which I took one of the summer volunteers with me. Paul had been born with cerebral palsy; he staffed the Visitor Center desk and had a signature joke for the tourists—that he was built like a buffalo: big head and shoulders, tiny legs. He walked with forearm crutches, dragging his legs along *scruff scruff scruff*. I will tell the truth and admit I had a speck of resentment for his presence: his weakness was bound to tax the rest of us, someone had to put his shoes and socks on in the morning and take them off again at night. When a male ranger was assigned this task, I was relieved. The intimacy of holding someone's foot in my hands terrified me and made me think of the apostles and Jesus, how all that footwashing created a sexual quantum field when I read about it on Wednesday afternoons at the Catholic school.

On our trip, Paul paddled strongly and we laughed. But when we returned to the boat ramp, I could not lift him out of the kayak to stand with his crutches. So I dumped him out, and that worked well enough because he could use the water to buoy himself up, though afterward I insisted on going to the grocery store, since the lake was halfway there, and I made Paul wait in his wet clothes while I went shopping, despite his shy complaints. My impatience mortifies me when I think back, now that I'm the one who's always slow.

Sorry . . . sorry . . . this is a song the Subaru's tires sing.

As we rise to the lake, Becky tells me about the time she herself climbed Mount Rainier, when she was a student of Willi Unsoeld's at the state college in our town that was founded in the 1970s as an "alternative" institution. Unsoeld is a legend there, a philosophy professor and a mountain climber. Becky says that she climbed as one of the students tied to Unsoeld's rope when he led a mob of them to the top in 1972. This is a poignant story because Unsoeld died a few years later while leading a student group down from the summit in a storm. One student died also, and Becky was asked by Unsoeld's widow to call the girl's mother. We speculate that she made this odd and too-intimate request to prove he was not a reckless man when it came to shepherding young people through the wilderness.

I'll say it again: many of us can be made bold by grief.

But grief can only transform the actual body so far, and our widower turns out to be trembling and pale-cheeked when we pull off just past the lake. We stop at a garden of creatures made from scrap metal, sculptures whose style resembles that of the driftwood fish and horse erected on the dry bed of the lake. Angus did not attach the windshield to his motorcycle, nor did he wear his leather jacket. When we ask why not, he gets a hangdog look.

"I wanted to look studly," he says, sucking in his belly. The thought had not occurred to me, that he'd seek romance on this trip. The day does not seem conducive to romance—the cloud ceiling high but solid.

The place called *Paradise* where the asphalt trails do their zigzagging lies at an elevation of 5,000 feet. His teeth are chattering but Angus assures us: "Don't worry, I will make it up to Paradise."

It is difficult for me to believe that almost twenty years have passed since I worked at the mountain. As soon as we go through the entry gate, I am ransacked by my old ghosts. We're in old-growth forest now, in the deep shade where the tree trunks glow reddish, almost purple, thickly grooved in patterns according to their species. We go by the limbless snags that are the remnants of a mudflow on Kautz Creek and by the trailhead of the secret trail I remember leading to two humongous Douglas firs. When we come to Longmire, the little enclave where I once lived, I am glad the place is more developed, bustling with people and tour buses. This little bit of ruin makes the sight of it easier to bear.

After Longmire, the angle of the road increases as the trees begin to shrink. We pass the trailhead to Comet Falls, which is the trail I took to my old workstation. I tell Becky about the man who tried to walk across the top of the falls in golf cleats, and about how his girlfriend ran all the way down to Longmire, out of her mind with the sight of his body dropping inside the water column. Marianne Moore wrote a famous poem about Mount Rainier, in which a mountain goat's eye is fixed on a waterfall "which never seems to fall / an endless skein swayed by the wind, / immune to the force of gravity . . ."

But of course the man was not immune.

The alpine meadow above Comet Falls is where I worked one summer, changing the signs (this is harder than it sounds, as they were planted in concrete) and repairing the trails. I tell Becky how Jim, back in the early days of our romance, came to visit me here in the rain. He'd hiked with two friends who looked hypothermic, so I made soup on my camp stove and saved the day—that's the kind of girl I imagine I was, the spunky saver of the day. We all weave our private myths.

Becky tells me that I'm still an Amazon, but I suspect she is just trying to make me feel good, seeing as she has a habit of overestimating human nature. These days I am a Roman, right there with Ovid when he says: *Call no man happy until he is dead and buried.*

Yet the challenge remains that there is still *this day*, which has erected itself before us like one of those signs planted in concrete. And I probably will live through it, a day when my friends and I are going to travel a mountain path, and we probably will see a bird or two and a flower or two, and those things should be goddamn good enough for me to record on my list of gratitudes.

Soon the Nisqually glacier appears before us, its snout like a strip mine, a pile of dusty slag filling the wide canyon where the glacier drips to form a river that is always being born. A wide steel bridge spans this place, a bridge that looks like it was built for the sole purpose of being ridden over on a new Harley-Davidson Dynaglide. I bet Angus is terrified.

In Marianne Moore's poem, this mountain is an octopus of ice, seen at first from the two-dimensional view of the map, the mountain outlined by the twenty-eight glaciers that sprawl down its sides. She wrote the poem after coming here on one trip from New York to visit her brother who was stationed at the shipyard in Bremerton. Her approach took a primitive version of this same road, as she too headed for Paradise.

The poem renders the mountain from varying perspectives—we see the rocks close up and from afar, we see both the map and the living mass. Moore quotes from a dozen sources, from spiritual treatises to tourist brochures, and we're referred to Henry James and Greek antiquity by way of explanation. She means to make us dizzy, as the colors of the lichen-covered rocks are dizzying: "the cavalcade of calico competing / with the original American menagerie of styles." The poem emulates in form the myriad stuff it is describing.

Filmmakers came to the mountain when I worked here to shoot some footage to accompany Moore's poem for a PBS series. As the resident ranger-poet, I lobbied heartily to escort them around the park. They too were from New York, and I remember their brand-new pack boots and enormous cache of M&Ms, as if they were prepared to bivouac for days. Their gear was hardly broken in, I noted smugly, before marching them straight uphill.

They needed footage to accompany two passages in particular, and my heart went haywire when they left the locations up to me. They wanted to illustrate the penultimate stanza of the poem, where Moore describes the trees she must have seen on her hike to the ice caves that once lay under the Paradise glacier:

Is "tree" the word for these things
"flat on the ground like vines"?
    some "bent in a half circle with branches on one side
    suggesting dust-brushes, not trees;
    some finding strength in union, forming little stunted
        grooves

their flattened mats of branches shrunk in trying to
     escape"
from the hard mountain "planned by ice and polished by
     the wind"

"Cushion krummholz" is the official name for these trees
stunted by the altitude, a term that is uncharacteristic of
Moore not to have used. The natural history contained in the
poem is actually a little crackpot, since Moore had also visited Banff on her trips west and conflates these two locations.

The filmmakers also wanted footage to suit the poem's
close, where Moore's version of nature gets wilder and more
fearsome, finally resulting in an avalanche going off "with a
sound like the crack of a rifle, / in a curtain of powdered
snow launched like a waterfall." So I took them to a place
where we looked down on the Nisqually glacier, the same
glacier whose snout we crossed on the road. (I think Moore
might have climbed down to it—there is a picture of her
standing on the edge of a dirty crevasse.) One of the sound
technicians threw a rock while the other held up the micro-
phone. And the result was strange karma—way across the
valley, as if in response, a small avalanche tumbled down.

Moore spent the night at the Paradise Inn, which is where
we go to take the chill from Angus's bones when we finally arrive at the top of the road. Built in 1917 in typical Park Service style, out of the kind of logs that epitomize Park Service
structures, logs that look as if they would make a good
throne for an ogre, the inn is a place where I rarely set foot
back when I was a ranger, meeting its comforts with my disdain, intended as they were for tourists, a word I always ut-

tered—like the other rangers—with derision. Becky and Angus buy chili at the snack bar, but I stick to the cheese I've brought and a mealy apple from my own tree. I can at least be a climber in this regard—eating bad, cold food.

From here, Moore hiked with her brother to the mountain's famous ice caves under the Paradise glacier, formed by the river that runs underneath. I do not know if Moore toured the caves as I did, entering the darkness with my headlamp where the river flows beneath the glacier, following the river until it exits at the wide mouth of the cave. Her poem is full of colors that seem accurate enough: emerald and turquoise and manganese-blue. They would have been lit by daylight through the dense quartz layer of the ice, which gives the colors a muted neon glow.

But the Paradise glacier is just about gone now, its lower reaches reverted to *firn*, the intermediate state between ice and snow. It is sad to fathom how the fundamental thing— a glacier—on which Moore built her poem could have disappeared, for the poem is nothing if not a statement about the endurance of the unfathomable complexities of nature in the face of the human desire to get them figured out. The fact that the glacier has melted away delivers a blow to the gut of the poem. It may have been complex, but it did not endure.

A few relatively flat meadows exist in Paradise—hence its popularity with nineteenth-century campers. From here a series of hillocks stair-step up—to a large snowfield that ends in Camp Muir, at 10,000 feet, where a climber has to rope up to begin glacier travel. On this day I can't see the mountain's top, and the high clouds shrink the distances. The Tatoosh Range is visible to the south—black crags down which I glissaded every summer, an unmarked route that dropped back to Longmire.

Today we set off to wherever the dinky concrete trail leads. You can tell that the ground is not used to being exposed, as it is on this dry year with scant snow cover—the soil is brown and dusty between the various clumps of alpine leafage. Angus keeps forgetting that it's against the rules to wander off the trail—whenever we see a flower his impulse is to march straight for it. I would prefer that no one talk, a remnant from those days when I traveled alone, but how do you say to your friends, *Please do not speak*? It is rarely possible nowadays for me to replicate the experience of traveling alone. Sometimes Jim and I can manage it, but I am tired of requiring a husband.

People coming down the trail nod to encourage me a little more enthusiastically than seems natural, but I will not let this piss me off today. The ones who keep to themselves are those who have come down from the mountain's upper reaches. When I worked here I climbed to the top each year, just to prove that I could, and so I know them not just by their plastic climbing boots but also from their leathered skin that tells me they have spent time above the clouds. You climb at night, when there is less danger that ice will melt and crevasses pop open, and you try to time it so that you get to the summit not long after the break of day. That first light is an oozy purple with the clouds below, when you gradually step out of their last stratum. That light is what people climb for, I think. Everything else is dark or heat or cold or exhaustion, but the early light is heaven.

Now there is one young woman walking down alone with ski poles in her hands to break the impact on her knees. Her hair has been pinned up carelessly, and her gaiters and clothes are ragged. I want to stop her and suck her blood: *I was you, make me you again.* I should know better—if she really is me, then she would probably resent the intrusion on her privacy.

Since I can't march, my plan is to be content with identifying the plants, even though it seems unnatural to wrench knowledge from the field guides without balancing that knowledge with some gained by experience. So I tell myself: *Okay, have an experience.* Two ravens swing on branches overhead along with the other birds made bold by years of snack food. This is my experience: to hear the ravens croak. To hear the slow, sporadic way they say the word *grok.* (This, the book says, is how you tell them from crows.)

It turns out that we are indeed late for the peak blooming weeks, which come right after snowmelt. And it is my habit to sulk when I feel that my perfect experience has been foiled by my disease—if I were healthy, I would have come here alone and sooner. But Becky points out that there are still plenty of ragged stragglers, like the blue cascade asters everywhere. And purple gentian, the last bloomers, just coming up, their flowerheads like little boxing gloves punching upward from the ground.

Dirty white mops, which are the seed heads of spent anemone flowers, stake the hillside. And the tall dry stalks of hellebore, a plant distinguished by its pleated leaf. Becky and I stop often to consult the field guides and play our knowledge game. Angus is fidgety and wanders ahead until he realizes he's lost his $500 Harley-Davidson sunglasses and heads back down in a tizzy to see if he's left them on the bike. We wait for him at a dip with a trickle of snowmelt where neon-pink monkeyflowers still bloom.

Even before he returns over the rise, we can hear him coming back up: now he's wearing the sunglasses and talking on his cell phone. When he gets off the line, I grouch at him for trammeling on my nature experience with his technology and loud blabbering.

"But I wanted to call my brother George! I wanted to tell him about all this!" His excitement shows in his voice's high pitch, as if we have taken him to the moon. He tried to come here once with his wife, he says, but heights scared her and they turned back.

And now my friends force me to turn back because the asphalt is getting rugged and ripped. I have no choice but to let them have their way since they are the ones who've been pushing me free when my wheels spin, though not to end somewhere spectacular seems anticlimactic, and I feel my expectations plummeting again, which forces me to find an Indian paintbrush flower still in bloom so I can write this down in my book of gratitudes.

The scooter skids down the pavement—the paths have been steeper than I realized. Angus and Becky walk in front of me and promise they're willing to throw themselves in my path if I lose control. I've given up on having a meditative experience, though there are not many people out on this gray day. Still, when we come to a marmot near the trailside, I tell my friends to shut up for a while.

The marmot makes a show of chewing its dry weeds, its silver fur rippling on its perch on a rock. Long ago, I chose this species for my totem animal: for its sweet whistle but mostly for its sluggishness and love of sleep. It does not keep score of its accomplishments. And it doesn't need to keep a book of gratitudes because it's grateful for every leaf it bumbles on.

We stand frozen, and the marmot doesn't flinch, not even when a family comes noisily trooping down the trail.

"Hey!" they yell to us, and still the marmot doesn't spook. "He was in that same spot hours ago when we passed him going up."

Marianne Moore also includes the marmot in her poem, supposedly as a surrogate for her brother, after learning that her first choice, the badger (from *Wind in the Willows*) was not found on this mountain. The marmot's whistle she describes as "the best wild music of the forest," the marmot itself the victim of "a struggle between curiosity and caution."

But our real marmot does not seem to be struggling with caution, and the only way we'd arouse its curiosity is if we held out a potato chip, which is against the rules. Moore quotes with condescension from the park rules of her day: "that one must do as one is told" and conform with the man-made regulations if one is planning to conquer the wilderness, the place where you'd think you'd be most free. Nowadays the most pointed example I can think of is that once you step onto the glacier to begin your travel there, you must carry down any waste you generate in a blue plastic bag. There are two methods, I was told: you either use the bag like a mitten or squat over it, making a direct deposit.

Two-thirds of the way through Moore's poem about Mount Rainier, she suddenly brings up the ancient Greeks and their fondness for smooth and polished surfaces, their shunning of the disorder that more truly characterizes nature. Happiness is attained by willpower, she says, with Greek civilization

> ascribing what we clumsily call happiness
> to "an accident or a quality
> a spiritual substance or the soul itself,
> an act, a disposition, or a habit
> or a habit infused, to which the soul has been persuaded,
> or something distinct from a habit, a power"

Happiness comes through persuasion and practice, according to Moore: it's an unnatural state of being that we can learn. As far as my own happiness goes, the first thing I have to learn in order to attain it is how not to envy healthy, hearty people like Marianne Moore—who poses in old photos with her gaiters and alpenstock.

The trip home was uneventful. Angus must have been even colder going down. At one point, as we drove the mountain road, the summit of Mount Rainier appeared through a hole in the clouds, a sight we had not seen all day. But when we pulled over, Angus signaled wearily for us to drive on. And a few days after our trip, he told me that as he shined the bike's pipes and tightened its bolts, he realized he'd become indifferent to it. The motorcycle was just a surrogate, he realized, when what he really wanted was a woman.

(Sure enough, by the time I edit this, the woman is found and the bike is sold.)

As for Marianne Moore, I was surprised to read that on her second trip west she didn't even go to Mount Rainier. The mountain wasn't what she wanted, though I don't understand it—how a healthy woman could *not* want the mountain. But she was content to study it from a rented cabin sixty miles away as she devoted herself to the geography she was most passionate about, which was the landscape of her poem.

Fear of the Market

Because I grew up while Vietnam burned, outside the garden walls of my young brain (a lot of hormone molecules in there, with carbon chains tangled like vines), I'm embarrassed to admit that for a while I was a cheerleader in high school. By chance I'd discovered I was good at jumping with my spine bent in an unnatural curl—people gasped at its severity. This caused me to experience, for the first time, the head-rush that results from getting admiration from one's peers, a feeling that is not wholly pleasant to me, yet I have repeatedly chased after it.

We wore home-dyed panties underneath our skirts, their washed-out green color inspiring some magical thinking that they were not underwear after all. Once I absentmindedly jumped in plain white ones—to hoots and giggles. For the rest of the practice session I only simulated the jumps by rising from a squat in a bizarrely constrained way, swiveling one saddle shoe in a frogish kick.

To raise money for new wool jumpers, Miss Cropsey decided that we would sell Christmas candles, little votives whose holders were covered in red or green velvet with fake pinecones attached. We all received a box of samples and an order form: we were to lug the box from door to door. The road in my neighborhood was winding, its houses far-flung gothic structures in many of which I had never spied a human form. This absence left me free to imagine who lived there. And since the very idea of salesgirlship fueled my apprehensions, I drew customers from my worst dreams. I feared they'd take it as an insult if I tried to fob Christmas off on them. Their celebrations probably featured a goat instead of Jesus.

Indeed, the hags and warlocks were not interested in my wares (actually the only people I made contact with were cleaning ladies), and after some halfhearted dragging of the sample box along our desolate suburban road, I brought it home and stored it in the closet, from which it spoke from time to time as the weeks went by. It sat in the closet's must and dark until the due date came for the order form, when my mother bailed me out by ordering three of each style of candle. And so for the remainder of the time I resided with my family, my failures were dug out each year and used to decorate the house. Over the years the velvet snagged more and more dust, until the merry colors turned to gray.

This is how it goes for introverted kids—whether we're talking Christmas candles or Girl Scout cookies. Now when I see the Scouts staged at the post office exit, I wince on their behalves, though I notice that these days there is always a parent dispatched to mastermind the ploy. The adult launches the girls toward likely marks after having whispered come-ons into their ears. This sort of shilling works because it is embarrassing to all involved, and we'll gladly pay the bribe so as to suffer through only its briefest form. And usually there is one girl who hangs back, clearly ashamed of the commerce in whose service she's been charged to lend her body.

She is the one I buy my Thin Mints from.

What I really want to talk about is my attempt to sell my book of poems, an art form I've been practicing for long enough now that I can't really speak of humiliation memories but rather . . . what? Humiliation loci? Nodules? What I mean is that humiliation turns into an ongoing, inhabited state because writing itself is of this nature. It's the flagrant narcissism that's so humiliating—writers think their creations are worthy enough to be circulated and admired; they secretly harbor the pride of new parents who are annoying in their certainty that, out of all the universe forged by procreation, their own child rises above the rabble. Then print serves to cast one's vanity in cement.

This is why some writers, like Emily Dickinson, avoided publication, which she famously called "the Auction / Of the Mind of Man." She left her poems in a drawer, but only after meticulously copying them out and sewing them into pamphlets. That such care went into their presentation suggests she was carefully orchestrating her legacy—and that her ego was big enough to lead her to assume that she would *have* a public legacy. Though she withdrew from the world, her arrogance was still stupendous.

Dickinson's lines announce that she pooh-poohs publication—or at least assumes the pooh-pooh pose—so as not to be soiled by poetry's commercial aspects. For even if no money changes hands, the poet incurs a debt through publication. Publication is an anti-barter, a negative exchange, so eager are poets (Dickinson included, at least early in her writing life) to be published that we are willing not only to give away our work for free but also to become beholden to whoever will disseminate it. The Internet has lately democratized this transaction by making publication available to all. This shifts the poet's debt from publisher to reader, the desire for publication being easily satisfied. Instead, we are in debt to the reader's time and attention, more than ever now that the whole world is reciting round the clock via weblogs and electronic "zines."

In Dickinson's day, poems would appear in the local paper—they were not just the froufrou artifacts of a fringe subculture. But no longer is poetry considered an appropriate companion to the spooning-up of oatmeal, and poets receive many signals from many different quarters that their work is trivial. More correctly, I should say that, though some types of poetry are bestowed with a large value by our present culture (I'm thinking of popular song lyrics and the spoken words we could corral under the heading of rap) (of course there will always be debate about whether these forms qualify) (I mean qualify as "literature" though I don't know exactly how I personally would draw the Venn diagram for the sets "poetry," "literature," and "song"), what has lost its cultural worth is the kind of print- and page-directed arrangement of words that expects a sustained engagement from its reader. When this kind of poem is read out loud in book-stores or college lecture halls, the environment created is un-like any natural one except maybe a Unitarian church service.

If looked at without any romantic attachments to the art, one might say that this kind of poetry has a negative value in the esteem of most citizens. Were even the most idiotic real-ity TV show to be interrupted by a public broadcast of T. S. Eliot reading *The Waste Land* (recently voted—by poets—the greatest poem in English of the last century), mayhem would ensue. I've seen many eyes glaze over when some fes-tivity is kicked off by the public reading of a poem, and even members of my own family will not come to hear me read. To be charitable, let's say they stay away because they're afraid I'd bore them, and they do not wish to break my heart by drifting off to sleep.

My embarrassment about being a poet comes partly from the narcissistic aspect of publication but also partly, I confess, from poetry's having so little value in the marketplace, my brain possessing a tiny lobe that desires economic rewards. My father was always mystified when he phoned and asked what I was doing and I answered that I was working, work being something you get paid for. When the Lilly drug com-pany heiress left her money to *Poetry* magazine, my mother, like many other Americans I'm sure, felt that it would have been more conscionable for the money to have been given back to all the people who were overcharged for their drugs.

My parents' trouble stems from the fact that the value of

even the most famous poems cannot be assessed, their worth being nil to much of our culture partly because their medium, language, is so ephemeral and cheap—and has been suspect almost as far back as its inception for being capable of pulling the wool over our eyes. In the past, sometimes an advertising agency would glom onto some fragment of poetry's high rhetoric—this happened to T. S. Eliot's lines "Time present and time past / Are both perhaps present in time future" (which were used to sell cars) and also to W. H. Auden's "We must love one another or die" (which was used to sell the nation LBJ). But lately our culture has lost its habit of respecting instances of graceful speech. It has been almost forty years since we've admitted lines from orators like John F. Kennedy and Martin Luther King into our daily conversation.

Usually poetry proves too elusive to be of much use as a commodity. By way of example, because it's short, I'll use the famous poem, originally an untitled section of a mixed-form book-length work by William Carlos Williams, that goes

so much depends
upon

a red wheel
barrow

glazed with rain
water

beside the white
chickens.

On the Internet I find that a rare-book dealer is asking $2,500 for a signed first edition of *Spring and All*, the book in which this first appeared, but of course it is the paper itself that wears the price tag. The value of the poem itself can't be assessed, unless we could figure out how many people have been employed teaching it, or we calculated the other subtle social functions of the poem—like how many teenagers read the poem and decided to become writers instead of petty criminals (though in one survey, college freshmen reported that this was the poem that, having been forced to analyze it in high school, they hated most).

Even poets would concede that the actual words of "Red Wheelbarrow" are of little value in aesthetic terms. They are pedestrian, and most of them fall—with the exception of the verb *glazed* and the somewhat archaic *upon*—within the range of grade-school language. It is the mysterious equation set up by the first line that gives depth to the poem, which was little noted until a good thirty years after it was first published. It then won its throne because of how neatly it summarized the complex idea that not only helped create Ernest Hemingway (the idea insisting that complex ideas can only be rendered though concrete things) but also the painter Edward Hopper, who turned back to realism despite the twentieth century's abstract vogue.

The poem nudged the culture. How much is this worth?

In 1979 a poet named Lewis Hyde published a book called *The Gift*, which wrestles with the value of intangibles. (One section discusses the Ford Motor Company's calculating the worth of a human life as $200,725 in 1971 after the car named *Pinto* repeatedly exploded. More recently, the Department of Transportation has assessed a life at $3 million, though the Environmental Protection Agency calculates its worth at more like $6 million.) For its central project, the book tries to make a connection between poems and the gifts that many cultures, like the Native American tribes of the Pacific Northwest, exchanged as part of the annual cycle of living. Sometimes valuable gifts were also destroyed by their recipients, a gesture insisting that the gift was not to be converted to personal wealth.

Instead, the circulation of gifts cemented the tribe the way ions flowing through a magnet will bond other metals to it. Gift-giving was largely restricted to the confines of the tribe, who understood the rituals of the exchange. Outsiders didn't, such as when Native Americans gave the European settlers gifts with the expectation that these gifts would then be passed on, this circulation a mandatory aspect of the ritual (hence the origin of the expression *Indian giver*).

These ideas can easily be applied to the way poetry is received, here in the American now. Poets are said to be an insular tribe who exchange their gifts mostly with one another, the readers of poetry being poets themselves. (Though I did go to a yard sale last year where a woman recognized me from the picture on my book. "You must be a poet," I said, and she answered no, she just happened to read poetry. "So you are the One! The One nonpoet reader of poetry in the land!" I shouted. But from the way she rolled her eyes I could tell it was a familiar joke.)

A friend who is a scholar has pointed out that the ideas

sketched out in *The Gift* are very much in keeping with the anti-consumerist counterculture of the 1970s, and therefore come tinged with a sentimentality whose shelf-life has expired. Poets now occupy the middle class, by dint of the increased presence of creative writing in academia; yet while this explosion of interest has occurred, poems have continued to go extinct from general-interest magazines like *Rolling Stone*. My brain sometimes is hobbled, not so much by the depreciation of a poem's dollar worth as poetry's wholesale dismissal from the assembly of art worth attending to, and I have to talk myself into the idea that there is a value, a pseudo-monetary value, attached to the poem. Or that no-value is still a value, an anti-value that suits the anti-barter.

Native American cultures do provide useful metaphors to describe poetry's circulation, especially when it comes to the differences between trade within the tribe and trade with outsiders. Within the tribe, what is traded must belong to the realm of gift; commerce is restricted to strangers. Among poets, monetary transactions often come off as tacky when they're made with other poets. The most memorable example I can think of is contained in Rainer Maria Rilke's *Letters to a Young Poet*, the record of a correspondence he maintained for several years with a (slightly) younger man named Kappus. In his third letter, in response to what has apparently been a request for books, Rilke writes:

> Finally, as to my books, I would like to send you all that might give you pleasure. But I am very poor, and my books, once they have appeared, no longer belong to me. I cannot buy them myself—and, as I would so often like, give them to

those who would be kind to them. So I am writing you on a slip the titles (and publishers) of my most recent books (the latest, in all I believe I have published some 12 or 13) and must leave it to you, dear sir, to order some of them when occasion offers. I like to think of my books as in your possession.

This passage has always stuck with me because it is so obviously wrought from connivance. Rilke professes generous intentions and then flatters the sensitivity with which Kappus would hypothetically receive the books, all of this a buildup to the sales pitch and the come-on of "dear sir" before Rilke seals the deal with the confident assumption that Kappus will rush out and buy. We do not like to see our literary heroes in such a sniveling light.

This explains why it's extremely uncomfortable, for example, to maintain one's own cash box at a poetry reading where books are being sold—the poet makes someone else do it so that he or she will not be soiled by money. In actual practice, poets have always marketed themselves: in America, Walt Whitman set the template for unabashed self-promotion by almost singlehandedly producing his books, taking charge of all aspects of their dissemination, from printing to advertising to finally mailing orders out, and even reviewing. (His reasoning: "I have merely looked myself over and repeated candidly what I saw. . . . If you did it for the sake of aggrandizing yourself that would be another thing; but doing it simply for the purpose of getting your own weight and measure is as right done for you by yourself as done for you by another.")

Lewis Hyde calls "the labor of gratitude" part of the circular passage of a gift and maintains that this "is wholly different from the 'obligation' we feel when we accept something we don't really want. . . . Giving a return gift is the final act in the labor of gratitude, and it is also, therefore, the true acceptance of the original gift." But I see two stumbling blocks in front of this theory about how poetry circulates: first, what if the return gift violates the terms of the ritual in some way? A recent pointed example was Amiri Baraka's creating, in return for the state of New Jersey's mantle of poet laureate, a poem called "Somebody Blew Up America," which accused Jews of having foreknowledge of the destruction of New York's Twin Towers.

The second problem is more significant: what if poetry really *is* something most people don't want—what if they'd rather see advertisements for products they might use instead of the poems that civic arts organizations are always trying to foist on them on the city bus? How does this lack of interest transform the gift? Presumably, the Northwest tribes savored the food exchanged at their feasts. But what if you brought a bowl of silkworm larvae to a modern-day potluck supper—nutritious food that is even considered a delicacy in some parts of the world? I bet you would have a hard time getting people to eat the larvae. Or if they did, it would only be because eating them would prove their macho fearlessness.

When my book of poems went out of print, I bought half the copies that were to be destroyed—seven hundred—for a dollar and nineteen cents each. I'd read about other writers doing this, a truck arriving with pallets that required a fork-lift, but when the shipping line's semi finally pulled up in the alley and the driver hoisted up the roll-door of the trailer, my heart deflated a bit when I saw only a stack of cardboard boxes, half the size of a refrigerator, strapped in the rear of the empty truck. The boxes looked sad in their grimy cavern, like a dwarf wearing a grown man's shabby tuxedo. Where could he be going, dressed like that?

Answer: to my storage locker, a warren of rooms made from plywood behind the bus station downtown. Not having any windows, the place was pitch-black when the lights weren't ticking around their timers for a maximum of fifteen minutes, after which the lights clicked off again to leave me stranded in the dark. Without delay, I made a stab at selling some books. I took a few over to Barnes & Noble, where the clerk summoned a manager who said they could only sell books that were provided by their corporate headquarters in a city far away.

But I live here, I said. I'm local.

Sorry, they said, you don't have a vendor number. Any-thing we sell has to have a number. Then I said, *Well then per-haps you would be interested in these candles. The velvet is dusty but they are brightly colored underneath.*

The local used bookstore took a few, however, and even treated me kindly enough to pull me from my dejection flash-back. But I knew it would take at least a century for seven hun-dred copies of my book to dribble from that store. So I took out an ad in a review where some of my poems were going to appear, a friend having sketched it up on her computer.

It was a small ad that cost eighty bucks, but when the review dropped through my mail slot a few weeks later I was stunned to see it enlarged to fill half a page. *We had extra space,* the editors said after I wrote to them in panic, *so we gave it to you.* That's how I learned one more thing about the taint of poetic commerce—the humiliation attached to it increases in direct proportion to the amount of space utilized for its purposes. A billboard might be a suitable place to sell a movie, but to sell a book of poetry it is unthinkable. Something about the proportion—little book, big ad—is painful.

This pain comes, I think, from the violation of the rules surrounding the circulation of gifts: the poet is supposed to say modestly to other members of the tribe, *Oh here, just take it.* Friends had stopped by when the books first arrived, and I'd told them that since I wanted to be rid of the books I was going to sell them for the postage cost. "Don't do that," they advised, "people do not value something if it costs them nothing." So they cooked up a price they thought appropriate. And it was thrilling, I must admit, when checks started appearing in my post office box, even though the thrill came tinged with shame.

Only one order came from a poet whose name I knew. Her tone was aggressively interrogative, wondering just exactly who was selling the books. "It's only me!" I wrote back—though she had a right to be indignant, being a midcareer sort of poet, like me, a member of the tribe with whom my trade ought to have been as gift. And my husband asked if I worried about cheapening myself. (Exactly what does it mean, "cheapen myself"? We do not want to be our mere

Ford Pinto versions. But I'm already a Ford Pinto sort of person, given to breakdowns and liable to explode.)

Poets generally delude themselves into thinking they are not selling anything, though books are objects to be sold, no escaping this base fact unless we throw our pages into brooks, as the great haiku writers of ancient Japan supposedly did. There's also a blind spot in thinking about poems as being offered completely free, and that blind spot is—*oh, right*—posterity. Though the two poets singled out in *The Gift*—Ezra Pound and Walt Whitman—never made much money, both did obsess about the long haul and massaged their legacies in the most P. T. Barnum-esque ways. For one's poem to catch enough wind to get blown into the future: this is the biggest of the bucks, the ultimate payoff.

Yet the boundary between gift and commerce can sometimes be wiggly, like when I gave more copies of my book to the used bookstore (because they're sold out, success making commerce a smidgen less awkward) in exchange for store credit. And my encounter with the yard sale–hosting poetry reader also gives me the idea that I might have to rearrange my thinking about who comes from my tribe and who is a stranger. Indeed, various efforts have been made recently to pound a few holes through poetry's garden wall. One was undertaken by the former laureate Robert Pinsky: nonpoets were videotaped reading their favorite poems. These videos were then digitally archived and broadcast on public television (although public TV itself is an insular, some might say hoity-toity, world).

And here Lyndon Johnson returns to haunt us, in the

form of his boyish press secretary, Bill Moyers, who has produced documentaries about contemporary poetry, again for the viewers of public TV. I taught for the first time at a summer writing conference shortly after the first of these shows were broadcast, and the other (more famous) poets dismissed the way they thought their art was being milled to pabulum for the public. Using *The Gift* to analyze their response to Moyers's efforts, I might say they felt threatened by the way that tribal membership was being opened up to outsiders.

Other wall-holes have been punched by the American Poetry and Literacy Project, which has left thousands of free poetry books in public settings. Its catalyst was Joseph Brodsky, another former laureate, who wrote an essay that was delivered before the Library of Congress and later reprinted in the *New Republic*, in which he chastised America for letting its great poetry languish. "At the very least," he wrote, "an anthology of American poetry should be found in the drawer in every room in every motel in the land, next to the Bible, which will not object to this proximity, since it does not object to the proximity of the phone book." Later, this intimacy took a dimensional leap when the APLP caused poems to appear in the phone book itself.

Just as the human brain evolved with the talent of memory, it evolved with the capacity to forget as another survival trick. So I am quickly forgetting my vulgar attempt at sales, and I thought I would write about it before it slips from my head completely. All in all, I figure I sold forty books, and those I have left seem ripe for some sort of ecological building technique, as old tires have been used to make houses (once I rode on a plane next to a couple returning from a class about how to build these "earth arks," whose design had been pioneered by a forgotten TV star). I've also thought of giving the books away to try to rehabilitate the spirit of the gift, but I don't want to irritate the people who've already sent me twelve dollars. Plus, I have the sneaky and heart-crushing suspicion that I might have a hard time even giving away a poetry book.

Money is like sex in this particular American eddy in which we swirl. We post its icons everywhere, yet we do not consider it good form to talk about either subject in specific terms (as in the matter of tampons, our ads will never utilize the fine word *blood*).

As far as cheerleading goes, by my junior year I'd quit, because my "consciousness had been raised," as we said back then, and cheerleading had come to seem frivolous when so many pages of history were being written and college students were being gunned down by the National Guard on their baseball diamonds. Also, in those days it was not good form for cheerleaders to have hair on their legs, and I was letting mine grow in protest of the razor's tyranny.

KNOWLEDGE GAME: *Bats*

1

The bats slice through the neighborhood, over the food co-op on Rogers Street, navigating by the tallest trees. The sky has to have reached a certain color, all the egg-blue drained but the indigo not yet lit up: the bats emerge during the silver tones. They come from chimneys farther west, or from the cracks underneath loose shingles of the few old bungalows that remain unbulldozed up on Cooper Point. Most of them bypass the forest belt that drops eastward down the ravine, the trail there stair-stepped and impassable to me. Instead, the bats take the straight shot of the road, heading south, steering around the corner where Rogers makes a jog. They aim for the giant Douglas fir by the park bench that isn't there anymore because it was stolen.

That's where we wait, Sandra and I, a bit uphill, so we can see a big wide sweep of sky. But when they come—on schedule—the bats do not take this path of open air. Instead, they cut across a laundry line in the backyard of the stucco house with the roof curved like a saddle.

The big brown bats come first, flopping like large awkward moths. Then the little brown bats arrive in greater numbers, flying faster and with more grace. They turn ninety degrees into the alley as if they were traveling by map, sometimes at the level of our knees or heads. In the dim light, their bodies blur as they jerk up and down with each wing stroke—that's how you tell them from birds. Then they vanish down the alley like a gust of wind that came from a fire, specked with ash.

Sandra lies on someone's lawn, and I'm trying to figure out a comfortable way to use my elbow as a pillow as I look up from the wheelchair. I'm thinking about climbing down from it, so that I too can luxuriate as the stars sift their dust down. But I notice that she hasn't volunteered to help me up. The problem is that we met when I was young and she was middle-aged, and now I'm middle-aged and she is too old for such lifting. Time shuttles us from station to station like a train, and I wonder how it does the job so quietly, without the start-up moan and the screech of brakes.

In between corkscrewing my head up like a parrot, I look at the ground wistfully. Still no offer from my friend, whose getting old irks me, though she did identify every flower along Rogers Street to make sure I noticed it. How I irk her in turn is by never being able to accept what's presented as good enough. Rogers Street has thrown itself into one last gasp of blossoming, and Sandra's been trying to teach me the scientific names of ornamental flowers. The point of these knowledge games is: to have the *now* get large.

"But you can't know everything," I say as she does her lying-down while I twist my parrot-head. "Not even about one moment. Not every single species along the road. Not all the trees in the field of view."

"No harm in trying," she says from the ground. "As long as you're stuck in one place you might as well try to get to know it as well as you can."

I think, *Easy for her to say, her head resting comfortably in her knitted fingers.*

I think, *Come on, old woman, get me down, I know you can, I've seen you chop a cord of wood.*

2

How I've come to be looking at *this* particular tree and *this* particular alley is because last night I went on a nature walk led by *the bat guy*, who wore a fishing vest and a diamond earring. He carried a transistor radio–sized machine tuned to what he called the songs of the bats—the pinging of their sonar. Amplified through his machine, they sounded like kittens being drowned. The group of people who showed up was larger than he expected and gabbed while he spoke. I thought this might have irritated him, because later on he said that if we weren't seeing bats, it was because we were talking too much. Not that the noise would bother the bats—it was us who were too distracted.

This was down by the man-made lake at the center of town, where a cloud shaped like a falcon hung unmoving in the sky. I was glad for the chance to claim a sidewalk for my wilderness, between lampposts 43 and 44, just north of the bus stop. For a change, nature deployed itself in a spot that

I could access easily, though because of the road noise, most of the bat guy's introductory speech escaped me. I did hear, *Bats have no greater incidence of rabies than any other species.* When he takes them out of the nets when he's tagging them, he lets them bite his arm.

Then there came the usual crepuscular minutes when the darkness sneaks up and switches on, and that's when suddenly the bats came zipping between lampposts 43 and 44. They come to freshwater to feed on *midges mosquitoes damselflies,* I hear him say, and *nymphs emerging from the lake.*

Their shadows swatted our cheeks right there on the sidewalk; I could feel the whispery way they stirred the air. Despite my intentions, I shrieked, and maybe it was just my imagination, but I thought the bat guy gave me the stink eye, that I'd think the bats would be so dumb as to hit me. He says that if they can pick out a *moth* in complete darkness, for god's sake, they're not going to hit my head.

They hunt by sending cries into the world and gauging what's there by the speed with which anything comes bouncing back, and it amuses me to think we humans also operate in this manner, locating each other through the echoes of our screams (*bats are less closely related to rodents than primates,* the bat guy said).

Most of the group falls away when we leave the bus stop and cross from the lake to the upscale supermarket on the bay. The sky's gone fully dark now, and I think maybe people were scared by how swiftly and closely the bats approached, rabies or not. I try to imagine the soft unlikely smash of one colliding with my face.

From the waterfront parking lot of the supermarket, you can see the bats slipping around the sea wall on their way to the lake. They disappear into the black crescent between the bay at high tide and the concrete arch of the new bridge. We're gathered on the boardwalk that stretches along one side of the market, the bat guy using terminology like *the matrimonial roost.* Like *time expansion,* which means the way he can slow down the speed of his tape to make their screams sound more like chirps.

I write down: *screaming turns into chirping if you let time expand.* That's what happened to me, when I think of all the screaming I used to do whenever I thought about my future. Time expanded, and my screams turned into chirps.

3

Each night, they need to eat the better part of their weight in insects. With their wings unfolded, they are mostly skin, half pornography and half baby bird, and this leaves their bodies exposed to the night air, which means they need to eat a lot of calories. And so they eat to keep flying, and so they fly to keep eating. What we call a *vicious* circle.

4

A famous essay, "What Is It Like to Be a Bat?" was published in 1974 by a philosopher named Thomas Nagel. The essay is not so much about bats as about the problem of imagining

any alien consciousness. Nagel chose bats because they occupy a limb high enough on the evolutionary tree that they
clearly possess consciousness, and yet they perceive the
world primarily through sensory apparatus that's completely
unlike our own. Our attempts to define echolocation in
human scientific terms tell us nothing about what it's like
for a bat to be a bat. "Even if I could by gradual degrees be
transformed into a bat," Nagel says, "nothing in my present
constitution enables me to imagine what the experiences of
such a future stage of myself thus metamorphosed would
be like."

Since I'll never *know* what it's like to be a bat—I mean,
I'm not an idiot; I know I'll never know—Sandra and I are
free to pursue our game, which is not so much a knowledge
game as a child's game of imagining. Two women lying on
a stranger's lawn—no, that's wrong: one of them is simply
"parked"—trying to see bats, trying to imagine *bat-ness*. I
beam my thoughts into the sky, listening for an echo.

5

A week later, I'm at the matrimonial roost, out at the old log
dump on Woodard Bay: the trail here is an old road that's
been gated off, so I can wheel the mile to the water, through
darkening woods of sword ferns growing under the ancient
mossy trees.

What strikes me first, when I come out at the clearing by
the inlet, is the diamond moiré pattern of the surface, a

fishnet of black on silver that wobbles as the twilight flexes itself against the bay. Looking north, you can see where the inlet opens into bigger water, and the sky is lighter there.

The bats live under a trestle, on top of which a railroad used to run, hauling logs away after they were floated here by tugboat. Its boards weathered and splintering, the trestle has been surrounded by a tall barbed-wire fence from which "Danger High Voltage" signs now hang. At dusk the bats will fly the ten miles to town, where the freshwater in the lake provides a better supply of insects.

The bat guy happens to show up here tonight—I think he thinks I'm stalking him, though tonight he speaks to anyone who wants to listen. The bat club from Seattle didn't show up for their tour because the freeway was too backed up for most of them to make the drive south. The only person who got through is an older man whose eyes blink as though they're accustomed to a deeper dark, his pale hair tufted around his ears. He fiddles with his own bat detector hanging around his neck, as he tells me how the bats have sex in autumn but how fertilization of the egg is delayed until the spring. He shows no compunction about speaking of bat sex, even though I've come here with my friends' young boy and the vocabulary makes me blush.

He says it's a mystery, how the sperm are stilled. How the female lets them know when they're free, in spring, to storm the fortress of her egg. When he uses the word *hibernaculum* to describe the winter roost, this new word puts me into a heightened sensory state. I feel as though I've never seen such lilac-light before, or at least I've never so appreciated being in its presence, as the great blue herons croak from their nests in the trees.

When I ask how the bats carry bugs from the lake to their young here—I mean, do they carry the food like a plug of tobacco inside their cheeks?—the bat guys look at me like I'm a fool. Bats are mammals (well, of course I knew that). It shows me how much I've still been thinking of them as birds, regurgitating for their young. Instead, the three thousand females living here nurse their *pups* from their bat-breasts, after they emerge from hibernation and give birth—one pup per bat. The mothers need to eat their weight in insects to make enough milk, which is why they will make the long trip to the lake more than once each night. Little factories turning mosquitoes into milk. But I have trouble processing this information, hung up as I am on the idea of bat breasts. Twice as many breasts as pups.

The bat guys spar with each other in their own knowledge game, flinging around the terminology, the Latin names, *Myotis* this and *Myotis* that. They compete over numbers, who has seen how many bats of what species in what state in how many abandoned churches. I like the idea of bats being drawn to holy places (it makes me think of a drawing I've seen of Lucifer, looking like a hybrid of man and bat, caught at a sad moment, his wings drooping on the ground).

The two bat guys have a hard time speaking to us laymen because they have trouble gearing themselves down. I can almost smell their flywheels smoke, what with the friction between what they know and the version of it that the rest of us can understand. They tolerate us because they are so full of facts that they'll explode if they don't get the chance to eject some. But I think they aren't eager to let too many people in on the secret of this place, whose light would be ruined by too many spectators filling it up with chatter.

The silver of the water surface intensifies when the trees grow dark, and just when you think you might pass out if there were to be a further silver increment—that's when the bats begin to fly. The first one looks like a stunned bird moving in a daze above the picnic table and across the clearing. Long intervals come between them at first, but pretty soon time speeds up and bats start whipping through the air. We count to 250 in thirty seconds, the black threads weaving the twilight into a darker gauze from which the night is made. It takes maybe thirty minutes for all the bats to exit. In a squeaky voice, the child I've come here with reports on how he can feel his hair being lifted.

My last question for the bat experts is why the bats would choose a place so far from the lake, when there are many other abandoned piers in town because the timber industries that once ringed the waterfront have gone out of business. The bat guys say that no one knows; maybe it's the size of the cracks between the boards here. Bats like to squeeze into *not too large a crack*, they say; like animals about to be slaughtered, or like some autistic children, they feel secure when they're confined. Conversely, then, I wonder how vulnerable they feel when flying, and if this is why they restrict themselves by following such specific flight paths to the lake, after they stream in such precise columns from both sides of the trestle.

There's a diminishment that comes when the spectacle is through. How unbearable, this forced return to ordinary life. On the way back to the car, my friends' son holds the flashlight as we march along the road, the huge trees and the giant ferns invisible now. All we are is human, night-blind and wingless. Un-sonared. Then the night turns less than three-dimensional when the batteries in the flashlight die.

6

I was skeptical when the bat man told me to go down Rogers Street and look at *this* particular tree and at *this* particular alley, but here they are and there they go: flying toward all the nymphs waiting at the lake. Later that night, when all the indigo bleeds out of it, a woman comes barreling down the alley in her pickup truck, headlights off. She's gunning for a guy who's moving like a dustrag in the shadow of the privet hedges.

"Fuck you, you bastard," she says. "I'm going to kill you."

"You try to fucking run me down I'm going to call the fucking cops."

Their hollering echoes through the tidy yards, and what the world sends echoing back is a cop car. But its trajectory lacks the precision of the bats'. Instead, the cop swings too fast around the corner and almost crashes into another car. It's almost shameful—how, by comparison, our human choreography has so little grace.

7

When I went back to the alley another night, the man who owned the stucco house with the saddle-shaped roof came out to ask what I was doing out in his backyard. It occurred to me how strange a sight I'd be in the darkness, skulking. You lose many possible identities when you start to use a wheelchair, and skulker is one of them. But, on the positive side, I am not feared. This guy knows that since I can't climb his stairs, I cannot be a thief.

But he seems unsure. Perhaps he thinks the wheelchair's just a gimmick.

He tells me that the bats fly over his shoulders every night when he sits out on his deck. He's a hearty guy about my age, gesturing with his cigar. I explain how they use his alley as a route to the lake—isn't that intriguing, the *specificity* of their choice? How it's *his* alley that they prefer?

When he asks suspiciously why I'm so interested in bats, I take it as a code: *What is this rogue apparition doing in my alley?* My answer sidesteps him—I say only that I've been going on bat walks with the bat guy—because the answer is complicated, how I've been playing these games to plug the holes where I've been torn by what my Buddhist therapist calls the waterfall of jealousy and grief. How bats are supposed to make me not resent my friends who head off to camp in the mountains. The true explanation would take all night.

Pretty soon the bats have all flown on, and the home-owner, satisfied that I am harmless, snuffs out his cigar and retreats into the house. After that, it's just my brain alone with a crescent moon, which I see hanging over the school-yard when I climb back up to Rogers Street. It's the kind of moon that makes me think of the scythe that Mr. Death's supposed to carry. Except, tonight, Venus shows up too and hangs inside the blade.

8

Three weeks later the bat guy convenes us once again. When first we gather, there's still enough light for me to write down *flying foxes* and *interpretation of the teats*. When someone asks about mating bonds, we're told that *bats are promiscuous*. I write that down and then remember how Dracula seemed so chaste.

(Scientists discover that promiscuous males that have the biggest testicles also have the smallest brains. But I read about this later, when the winter torrents bloat the rivers as well as the soil that should be holding up the hillsides but does not, the bats gone off to hibernaculums where the females incarcerate the tiny ticking bombs of their eggs.)

This time I ask the bat guy how come he's not afraid of rabies, my mother having sworn to a story about how a little girl died when a bat bit her in her sleep. Then he explains the reason for his bravado—he's already had the rabies shots, so he's immune. Good—I want the bats to be in some percentage rabid, some percentage dangerous, I don't want them to be too tame. Instead, I want risk to be tonight's blind date. For his part, I notice that the bat guy doesn't like to talk about his day job doing something boring for the state.

This time the bats don't slice through the group assembled between lampposts 43 and 44, even though we can see hundreds of them feeding on the lake when he shines his searchlight across the water surface. I'm disappointed, although on this night I've come to see them fly across the harvest moon, which rises directly above the Ramada Inn, full and crisp in its topography. Even without binoculars its bright mountains are visible, as well as its dusty-looking plains.

The bats hunt low on the water, but every now and again, looking through my binoculars, I'll see one silhouetted by the moon's low orange wafer, the bat flicking into the field of view for only an instant. Shocking more than eerie, because of how large it appears, its wingspan wide as the lunar surface. And because of how clearly I can see the skeleton that's wrapped inside the frail skin of the wings. For one moment the bones hang motionless, caught as if by strobe-light. The body saying, however briefly, *Here I am.*

Brief History of My Thumb

I remember how it felt to get into the car. This was the part I liked best, the part when I was a little afraid.

To the driver—who was usually a man alone—my eyes gave just a flicker. Sometimes a woman would stop and I knew what was coming: a lecture about the risk. She was trying to save me, and who knows, she may have. The next car coming along might have belonged to the psychopath who would have killed me long ago.

In the beginning, it was me and my high-school friends who entered the cars' sweaty interiors. We girls, and it was always girls, let ourselves be borne two miles up our town's one road. We got out, crossed the road, and repeated the process on the southbound side. The point was not to go anywhere. Then what *was* the point? The answer I leave to Heraclitus:

> The rule that makes
> its subject weary
> is a sentence
> of hard labor.
>
> For this reason,
> change gives rest.

Heraclitus was the one who said famously that you can't step into the same river twice. More precisely, he said (in Brooks Haxton's translation) that just as the river he stepped into "is not the same, and is, so I am as I am not."

A teenager likewise inhabits two states, grown and not, though I would have scorned anyone who identified me as a child. I was a match burning down to a black spindle. When I stood by the road, its ditch-wind fed me and made my little flame rise.

Later I moved not too far away from home, but to Quebec. I chose a foreign country to give my acquiescing to this conventional duty—going to college—a varnish of the exotic. I also wanted to escape my house where the televisions blared in every room and people screamed above them. The cars, by contrast, were calm places where I was almost always free to smoke cigarettes.

In Montreal, it seemed everyone smoked and everyone hitchhiked, because of a bus strike that went on for weeks. Beautiful women stood alone in the slush at the side of the road and stuck out their thumbs. I was sad to see the strike end and the sexy French women in their high-heeled boots suddenly disappear back to whatever swanky place they came from.

In my sophomore year I transferred to the agricultural college, whose buildings squatted in a wind-scoured pasture, flat as an airstrip, between two freeways. Quivering concrete ramps and roads led into the city thirty miles away. I cut my hair and wore a watch cap and down jacket, so that I looked like a husky boy. Dimly I was aware that I was acting out an archetype from old folk songs: that of the wife who goes to war or the pirate whose bound breasts are discovered after his death. When I stood at dawn on the elevated highways, the gusts of semis nearly blew me off my feet.

But in my youth I rode inside a bubble of luck: the worst thing that ever happened was that a man pulled out his penis. I started making up rules. Number One was to never look at the driver. Then he could have his penis out until the cows came home. Rule Number Two was not to get into cars with more than one man in them, because once, when I rode squashed in a car full of man-boys, one draped his arm across my shoulder, ostensibly to save space, and then let his hand droop until it touched my breast. Just the side, just through my shirt. He was daring me to scream. When I looked down, I found myself inappropriately dressed, as in a type of anxiety dream. I wore no bra, and the shirt's crinkly green cloth, I realized, had shrunk a bit and puckered around each button to reveal a half-dollar-size glimpse of skin.

Early on, I'd decided that it was a bad idea to call attention to the transgressions of the men, because then they might decide to hurt you. In my French gibberish I announced they'd missed their turn, and they believed me because they were unfamiliar with this part of the province. They let me out in a muddy strip between the speeding cars and the concrete barricade.

When I graduated, I went to live briefly on a farm in Vermont that was run by women, where one of my housemates made her living by crocheting vests and taking them to craft fairs around the country. Lucy did not own a car; few of the women on the farm had enough money or would have wanted a machine that was such an ecological scourge. So she sent her vests by mail and hitchhiked after them. When I asked about whether she was afraid of being raped, she answered that she had been, recently, and then of course I wanted to know why she still hitched.

"What I can't bear to give up is the feeling," she said. "Just me and my thumb all alone on the road." I said I knew what she was talking about. The immense spaces inside of which the hitcher becomes tiny. And the sudden diminishment is thrilling: *whoosh*. Small becomes big, and there you are, standing alone with Heraclitus again. Even rape didn't quash him.

But of course I didn't have a clue.

These stories came to an end when I bought a truck. By then the sentiment of the highway was changing anyway, so that no one of legitimate sanity picked up hitchers anymore. For a while I felt obligated to make the reciprocal gesture as payback for all the rides I'd been given, until more than one drifter scared me when I realized he had nowhere to go and wanted to attach himself to me. Then I had to scramble for an excuse to kick him out. I usually said, *you have to get out here, I'm turning back*.

Some of the ones I blew by still haunt me, like the Indian woman on crutches way out in the desert in New Mexico. She's wearing a bandana and she's crying. I think about turning around for her sometimes, but now it's twenty years too late.

And some of the ones I picked up still haunt me too, like the man-boy in Colorado who was traveling to an uncle who had promised him a job. He did not know exactly where he was headed, and so I tossed him the Rand-McNally road atlas. He flipped and flipped, from one cover to the other, until I realized that he couldn't alphabetize, could not read the word *Colorado* where it was printed in the corner of the page. He had the name of the town where he was supposed to be headed written on a scrap of paper, but could not pronounce the words. "Booey veh . . ." he muttered before finally handing me the scrap, on which I decoded *Buena Vista* spelled badly in the strange glyphs of someone who didn't know the alphabet.

Now, in the new millennium, we drive and make phone calls at the same time, and the car operates in sympathy with the clock. This is no country for backpacked young women: *You don't know what kind of river you're stepping into, I may never be the same, but that doesn't mean that I am good.*

I trade stories often enough with women my age, about our lives as hitchers, to know it is not an uncommon history, though *hitch* isn't a word we use anymore except in regard to knots. We've experienced middle-aged reentry, and we hunker now inside the nose cone that has returned safely (maybe), unraped (no—the other woman often has her rape story to tell, if she will tell it), as we bob in the sea. Heraclitus had nothing good to say about the state of being wet. Better to be a dry thing, he thought, ready to be kindled into flames.

But some stories can't help being soggy, as on one dusktime in New Hampshire, when I find myself in my man-boy costume. Lugging skis and a pack, I have just come from Tuckerman's Ravine, a bowl whose walls are famously steep, and I am feeling like an epic hero for having skied down them alone. This time, instead of mysteriously ending up half-clothed, I've just as mysteriously ended up on the road with too large a load. My thumb brings no luck as the sky turns black and sends down starlight only in the form of giant flakes.

Finally, a semi stops—its headlights bore a tunnel through the swirling globs of wet snow while I climb into its cab. The driver reacts with surprise when he realizes I am a girl, and for a while I try to talk to him in French, though in no time I fall asleep. It is a mystery to me, how we crossed the border—and I wake up slumped against him. My drool is cold and wets his sleeve.

Bonnie Without Clyde:
The Romance of Being Bad

The movie *Bonnie and Clyde* opens with Faye Dunaway wearing not a stitch—she's just a daybreak cloud in false eyelashes. When she looks through the bars of her iron headboard, we know this shot means to show us that she feels like she's in prison there in her mama's house. And also that her body is part of the prison problem, that she wants to make some kind of storm with its rosy cloud. The lightning will come from her tommy gun and the rain will be her blood. So the movie's violent final splatter tells us nothing we don't already know two minutes in.

The appeal of the clodhopper who is Warren Beatty's Clyde is that he intuits all this about her when he shows up out of nowhere to steal her mama's car. Good thing he's impotent, that instead of his penis he puts a gun into her hands, which suits her better anyhow, since she can be photographed with the gun as though it were her own lethal erection. And though the critic Pauline Kael was a fan of the movie, she faulted its cheesy climax, when Clyde is cured. What finally makes him hard (and though it may be cheesy, I do love this about the story) is Bonnie's writing a poem about him and then getting it published. To him, a published poem means bona fide (*boner-fied!*) immortality.

Kael points out that the movie's concoction of Bonnie is confused in the way it collapses time: the story takes place in the 1930s, but her makeup and hairdo put her in the 1960s, when the movie was made. If I think about an outlaw woman poet of the 1960s, the person who pops first into my head is Sylvia Plath, calling her daddy a bastard. This is a curious reversal: the child accusing the father of being illegitimate. It's a blasphemy that seems as ancient as it is screwball.

I remember vividly when my sister called my father a bastard. It only happened once, which gave the word special power to burn a permanent neural pathway in my brain. We-the-family were on our yearly Hajj to a whitewashed motel in Virginia called the Whispering Pines, a crumbling ruin, though the fame of its restaurant traveled miles. There, surreally dark-skinned waitresses served the soft-shelled crabs my father loved. Bonnie Parker happened to be what Pauline Kael calls a "waitress-slut," but the waitresses at the Whispering Pines were mythic, as formal as a Greek chorus, in starched white uniforms that sparked against their skin. In particular, I remember a woman in thick glasses who bussed the tables and wore a nametag that read I AM DEAF.

I should also mention that my father, whose frothing volatility masked his basic mildness, responded by slapping my sister's cheek. When I talk about this memory——the shy girl spitting out the curse and the ensuing crack-sound of the slap——my sister has no recollection of it. But I do, I swear, and because I'm the one writing this I get to control this version of the past, and I say that the bone of their contention was our daily outing in the Cadillac. On this day we were bound for the ferry to Tangier Island, a trip that my sister refused to take and so was hauled by force into the car.

In the end, she won because she got her wish not to ride the ferry: by the time we arrived, the boat had ceased operating for the day. Silently the six of us—or was it five? I don't remember my older brother's being present—rode back to the motel through the dead-flat countryside, with the air conditioning blasting and the Caddy's windows rolled up while, outside, the grass blazed up with the teardrop-shapes of flames. My mother kept us in line throughout the year by suggesting, at the climax of our battles, that we might move to this place. "A place that would be good for you children." We thought it shared the desolation of the dust-bowl countryside that Bonnie and Clyde rode through, and the thought of living there shut us up real quick.

Though it was the male poets of the last midcentury who first started writing autobiographically, it was the women who got slapped with the confessional label, which has come to mean a large degree of self-absorption combined with poorly edited melodrama. If one were to get paranoid about this, it might seem that the term *confessional poetry* was coined so that any eruptions coming from female quarters could be squelched. Sylvia Plath and Anne Sexton get singled out as the gun molls of the autobiographical/confessional gang, which has pretty much lost its male leaders, its Clydes—who ride now in a more luxury-class automobile of their own. Both Plath and Sexton were, however, influenced by Robert Lowell, who would make a very good Clyde indeed.

But Plath is not really a poet of social rebellion. She dons the roles of wife and mother willingly enough; although, granted, her take on these functions is peculiar, she doesn't necessarily resist them, except perhaps in her uncharacteristic poem "The Applicant," where a woman interviewing for the role of wife is instructed to wear a rubber crotch.

It is Sexton's poem "Her Kind" that ought to serve as a capsule of the feminist upheavals that were about to follow in the poem's wake (it was published in 1960). This is the early, formal, disciplined Sexton, and I have felt wronged by seeing it drop from the *Norton Anthology of Poetry* as Sexton's stock has fallen, perhaps because of the autobiographical Sexton's showboat qualities, which adhered to her poetry as her life burned on despite her attempts to extinguish it. In contrast to this aggrandized persona, the witch in the cart is archetypal:

> I have gone out, a possessed witch,
> haunting the black air, braver at night;
> dreaming evil, I have done my hitch
> over the plain houses, light by light:
> lonely thing, twelve-fingered, out of mind.
> A woman like that is not a woman, quite.
> I have been her kind.

That's the first stanza of the poem, perhaps a simplistic encapsulation of the isolation that many women felt in the suburbs after the Second World War (capsules need to be short and tart if they're to be carried around in the back of the brain). The poem puts its finger on the idea of *dreaming evil*, the primary operation of the female poet's outlaw fantasy life, a fantasy that served, in Sexton's case, as retaliation against life in the postwar suburbs.

In my observation, this fantasy past is created most often now by women who have chickened out on, or are recuperating from, our chance to hop in the car, and have instead become librarians and professors and schoolteachers and—oh worst—happy wives. In fact, we do not drink and fumble around in coatrooms with men, if we ever did at all, though we harbor the illusion that we did, along with the wish that we still lived in the days pre-AIDS, pre-hepatitis C and human papilloma virus and meth and crack and tweakers, in that narrow window of time—the 1970s I guess—when a lot of bad behavior was suddenly (thanks to the pill and penicillin) consequence-less. Fumbling around in coatrooms now comes off as merely self-indulgent, plus heterosexuality itself is a bit passé.

But the tradition of the female poet outlaw goes way back, as far back as Queen Elizabeth, who wrote, in 1589, a poem about how she wanted to chop off the head of her rival, Mary Queen of Scots. And even before this, in 1546, Anne Askew, who was arrested for heresy, wrote a poem that maintained her innocence and was burned at the stake for it. Rebellion is bad enough, but writing a poem about it doubles the crime. A poem is by its nature a public utterance, no matter how reticent the author, and to write one has always been an audacious act for women, especially when their poetry concerned extramarital love and civil war. So it makes sense that an audacious alter ego would have been created from the get-go, to carry the poem on its huge shoulders.

Later, among British poets, we get Aphra Behn's mid-seventeenth-century take on male impotency and women making love with women, and the globetrotting mega-outlaw (ditcher of husbands, taker of lovers, and introducer of smallpox vaccine to England) Lady Mary Wortley Montagu and her 1734 retort to her nemesis Jonathan Swift, in which she—speaking with the voice of a libertine persona who feels wronged by his inability to perform sexually—tells him that his poems will "furnish paper when I shite."

Now, in this moment: I pull poetry books down from my shelves until I assemble a big stack written by my more-or-less peers. Together we write this poem I call "Bonnie Without Clyde":

> I copped a .22 snugged in a black clutch bag,
> an ordinary woman who could rise
> in flame.
> God I was innocent then, clean as a beast in the streets,
> revved up on coffee, cigarettes, alcohol, the sound of my
>   own voice.
>
> It was almost biblical, driving the midnight burning
>   highway
> to a domed metal diner with seven red stools
> where the shadow pimps go *hey princess*
> (my mother's mouth still saying *Slut*).

People are afraid of keeping secrets between their legs
(I will be your naked doctor girl).
Those men I fucked when I was drunk: memory
is a little museum of miscalculation and haste.*

These lyric confession-outpourings are generally culled from the arenas of sex and crime, often related to drugs. But the mood that my Bonnies want to brew comes from Faye Dunaway's 1930s component, pre-dating the rock-and-roll music that would complete the famous trinity. The soundtrack of these poems would more appropriately be jazz, preferably performed by a tragic addict like Billie Holiday. For sure my Bonnies would not choose the movie's twangy bluegrass soundtrack.

Here is my crime confession: I once was a shoplifter of meat. Having been caught smoking pot by the women's dormitory resident (in Canada, these older students were called wardens*), my friends and I announced that we could not be thrown out because we were leaving, ha! The next day we found an apartment on a down-at-the-heels block of downtown Montreal, a city that barely functioned with all the chaos caused by the French separatist movement of the times.*

"Steinberg's" was the name of the grocery, and because we girls were

---

*This poem was made with the help of Kim Addonizio, Stephanie Brown, Denise Duhamel, Nancy Eimers, Amy Gerstler, Lisa Glatt, Lynda Hull, Dorianne Laux, Lisa Lewis, Suzanne Paola, Belle Waring, and Susan Yuzna. These poets share some similar subject matter though their syntax and diction, of course, vary.

poor—no, only pretend poor, it being part of the outlaw fantasy that we were not bred from the upper middle class—we felt as if we were being shadowed by a holy ghost who would both protect us from arrest and absolve the crime. It seemed outlandish that a person could get into trouble for stealing food (you see: I was such a dope I didn't even know about Les Misérables, whose plot is set in motion by the theft of a baguette).

I was not a member of the shopping expedition the week my roommates did get caught, one of them a basketball player who easily outran the store guard (since when had Steinberg's acquired guards?). The other captured roommate had a baby face and gave the guard the phone number of our apartment, where one of us pretended to be her mother. After being reprimanded, she was released. That night at dinner, buzzing with adrenaline, we all ate a celebratory roast that came out of the basketball player's purse.

When I wrote not long ago about fondling the giant purple slabs of beef, the thrill of slipping one into my purse, I realized that this writing was giving me tremendous pleasure, a childish thrill that came from conjuring my outlaw persona. It titillated me as I bent the real like a welder with a torch— had I ever stolen meat or had it been only the possessor of the baby face, the one who is now an oncologist in St. Louis? The oncologist who caused a strange woman to run up and give me an embrace, because my roommate saved her life?

In fact, I could have had all the meat I wanted, if I'd sacrificed my pride and asked my parents to send more money.

Unlike Bonnie Parker, getting something published has always filled me with shame, despite my having sought publication so avidly. This embarrassment may be congenital, my family having avoided leaving a paper trail that would cement us to any one reality. Had my grandfather come to this country by jumping ship in New York, or had he somehow made his way through Canada? And had his brother Stefan, also a sailor, committed suicide or been murdered at the docks? If I close my eyes, I can picture my mother's looping script, but my father's pens left the breast pocket of his suits only when he lost them. To shake my relations off my own trail, I considered using a pseudonym, like some of my friends.

Once when my parents visited me during the Christmas season, the three of us walked around Pioneer Square to look at the gleaming windows. They knew my first book of poetry was about to be published, and so they sent me into the bookstore to see if it had been shipped yet. And when I saw it standing on an end-cap, my breathing stopped and nothing in my body worked except whatever chamber of my heart it was that squirted so much blood into my face. I walked back outside into the snow (see how my memory embroiders the scene; the chance is slim that the clouds over Seattle could have actually dropped any snow).

"Was it there?" my parents asked.

"Not yet," I lied.

On this issue of whether writers should take the feelings of their loved ones into consideration when they wrote, William Faulkner counseled ruthlessness, saying that "Ode on a Grecian Urn" was worth any number of old ladies. This trade-off—family harmony versus heartfelt expression, once

I invented for myself a glitzier heart—worried me a great deal when I was young. Indeed, when my mother read my first book, after she'd spread the news of its imminent arrival, she remarked dryly/angrily/wistfully/shamefully: "I wish you'd told me what it was going to be like."

Question: What was it like? Answer: Full of much bad writing. I had too much investment in the autobiographical myth, which I thought was necessary because I lacked the inventiveness not to write about actual life, and I thought that actual life required a grand myth to be interesting—what could be interesting about a pasty-skinned girl from the suburbs? I hadn't gotten wise to Emily Dickinson yet, a poet who derived her outlaw spark from the sly rebellion of her strange punctuation. To put the brigand into the poem itself, not the autobiography, this is the harder trick.

Luckily, my outlaw period ended early. During that same freshman year in Canada, I hitchhiked across the border with a boy who taped six capsules of speed to his arm. How glamorous his long arm seemed when he rolled down his shirtsleeve and donned the leather jacket into whose pocket he'd forgotten to put his student visa. This was a boy who occupied a beauty tier that was at least one tier above my own beauty tier, and I thought my being as daring as he was would eliminate our visual discrepancy.

What I discovered from sweating out two hours at the inspection booth was that Thrill in general had outgrown me—it had become too large to inhabit my body without wearing it out. Plus a terrible disease (*a disease of the nerves!*) eventually took over as my life's master narrative. Though we were not strip-searched (allowed, instead, to return to the routine of our Monday-morning classes), I knew my life of crime was over.

Now that I'm feeble, I have the habit of revisiting it, if only through the lies that memory tells me as I sit here. From now on, I'll not easily be offered the opportunity to be bad. Or maybe the problem is that now I am too easily offered—forced to partake in!—the outlaw rituals of my youth. Drugs: I have many, lined up in the cabinet. Slothfulness comes easy to me, in my stony daze (800 mg gabapentin/ 4 times a day). My life has become not just tame, it transpires now almost *without event*, save for the drama of an accelerated physical decline. This physical dilapidation only makes the outlaw more cherished, seeing as she is so improbable. How could I rob a bank? Could I make my getaway in my rusted minivan? Every once in a while, I'll read in the paper about someone mounting this kind of doomed venture, and I can't help rooting for that old coot—it never seems to be a her—rolling away from the bank in a wheelchair while the ink-pack hidden in the money explodes.

Finally, if I may cut back to the movie, we see how a bald statement of the myth becomes the very thing that jumpstarts it, which happens early on, when Warren Beatty delivers his famous line to a dirt farmer who's gone belly up: "We rob banks." And so they have to go ahead and do this, to align the line with a life lived in accordance to its mythic promise.

The American female poets who've written The Famous Lines have lived lives equal to the great singularity of the lines, as if the autobiographical myth were a rocket booster for propelling the poet into history. The poet writes: *My life had stood a loaded gun* and becomes the recluse who will not let the doctor examine her when she is dying—he may only watch her pass back and forth across a doorway. Or she writes: *I eat men like air* and turns on the oven's gas. (*The art of losing isn't hard to master* also comes to mind, a line written by a poet impersonating a normal woman who rejected the grand autobiographical myth.)

As I sift both my brain and my *Norton Anthology* for such examples, I realize that we have not had enough years of female poets in this country to have a big stockpile of such lines yet. I mean the kind of lines that contain a tinge of infamy.

Sick Fuck

I began this by asking Jim if he'd mind being included in something I was planning to write about sex.

"No one wants to read about sex," he said.

"Everyone wants to read about sex!"

"Not about you having sex."

Then I had to admit he had a point. Ungrammatical as his response was.

Not about me, okay, there is nothing singular about me, my contortions are conventional—except that the puppet strings of my nerves have grown corroded with scar tissue. From a subjective perspective, this feels much as it sounds: my legs feel like the antennae of a TV tuned to a channel where no signal is coming in, and the static fuzz is humming loud. They've also become spastic, lock-kneed at odd moments, my feet like those of Barbie, ready for the high-heeled shoe.

It is not an appealing picture. But if I am going to write about my sex life, you should get a good look, especially at the segue from my legs to waist, where my body starts getting strange. I have had a machine implanted on my belly: it delivers drugs to my spine via a tube. The tube runs under my skin, and I can't feel it with my fingers except where it bends to enter one of the interstices of my vertebrae. The bend makes a spongy bubble in my back's lumbar curve, and when I first discovered this rubbery spot I could not keep from poking it.

The machine is about the size of a tuna can. Before it was implanted, the surgeon showed me how it looked: gleaming and pseudoliquidly silver, like my high-school track team's stopwatch. Its top side is flattened, which creates a point on either side of that flat spot where the metal feels to be just one cell-layer away from breaking through my skin. The surgeon whom even Jim calls Doctor Dreamboat (tall, handsome, flies plane, etc.) made a pocket under my skin and slipped the can into it like a large item zipped into a small coin purse, so that now it rests just forward of the wingbone on my right hip. A three inch scar runs above it, and because the incision did not close properly there is a dry purple lozenge of scar tissue at the center of the slice, where the incision puckers in, just above the place where the device's arc is flattened.

When I volunteer to show off the machine, men in particular usually turn down the opportunity, though it's a party trick in which I take some glee—if the body has to be defiled, one might as well spread the discomfort around a little. Only after the operation was I struck by the lightning bolt of sexual implications, having changed my frontal view forever. But this is how time iterates itself for everyone, I know, I know, by hacking us to bits—the breast removed, the kidney taken. This is the storyboard of the modern body. Or we are remodeled with added bits, with titanium under our skin or inside our arteries.

The pump and its scar fit exactly in the palm of my hand, with my thumb resting on the flattened spot. When I am trying to give an erotic purpose to my nakedness and do not have an appropriate piece of drapery, I leave my hand there like Napoleon with his wrist curled into a pocket.

Even though the disappearance of one's young body is a tired lament, it is especially galling to me not only because of how I once worshipped at the temple of physical fitness, but also because of the extremity of my body's being sacked. When I asked Jim the other day how he could stand making love to such a freak, he said: "That's what eyelids are for." (Of course, the word *freak* is somewhat confrontational, somewhat melodramatic in its assessment of the body, and in slang usage it also refers to a person who is willing to defy sexual convention. Which is another form of aggrandizement, this defiant persona used to fill a vacuum caused by the body's losses.)

So we keep our eyes shut, though actually the dropped lid was always my preference—I never wanted to see the face that makes the cry that poet Louise Glück calls "the low, humiliating / premise of union." Before her, Charles Baudelaire elaborated in prose, and at greater length, on the subject:

> Do you hear those sighs, those groans, those cries, those rattles in the throat? Who has not uttered them, who has not irresistibly extorted them? These unfocused sleepwalker's eyes, these limbs whose muscles spring up and stiffen as if attached to a galvanic battery: the wildest effects

of drunkenness, delirium and opium will certainly not give you such horrible and curious examples. And the human face, which Ovid thought was created to reflect the stars: there it is, bereft of speech, with an expression of wild ferocity, or slackening in a kind of death. For certainly I think it would be sacrilege to apply the word *ecstasy* to this sort of decomposition.

The face is embarrassing and also frightening: the body at its moment of utmost concentration, as if it were in the midst of committing a violent crime. But then also, oddly, the face looks almost bored, as if it is about to drop off into sleep, as if it were a decoy face we concoct to camouflage the oddity of what is going on. This is probably why female praying mantises chew off their mates' heads: so that they never have to see that face again.

Especially maddening is the knowledge that we are being looked at just as we are looking: in order to proceed, I have to make myself forget this, and then I soldier on alone. But when I close my eyes and conjure images, the merest whisper of disease will kill the romantic urge; so my real body must be banished, forgotten, in a fudging of the facts. To do the work of my delusion I call on what I call "the dirigibles," zeppelins made of skin, my surrogate inflatables—(that archetypal taut flesh)—from the planet of their silk bedding. From the journals of Anaïs Nin with their fringed lampshades and brocade pillows. From the cranial basement's leather chambers with its pneumatic apparatus.

When I was a kid, the inflatables were treasure, buried

under my father's mattress where I'd find not just *Playboy* but also higher-toned men's magazines like *Argosy*, which featured hoity-toity nudes photographed through colored filters. I remember bringing a copy to the storeroom of Mr. Phillips's fourth-grade class, where we girls—and only girls, as the boys did not seem courageous enough to invite—scrutinized the torsos that ultimately yielded none of their secrets despite the intensity of our interrogation. The secret of buttocks' rolling countryside and the nipple's artsy silhouette.

In my imagination, these surrogates are like elephant seals—the male-to-female ratio among their population is low—and possibly this is because of how they entered my childhood brain, as a girlish preoccupation. The bodies called like sirens, and the quest for them took me to my father's nightstand and through his drawers, then to tree houses and crawl spaces crisscrossed by sunlight coming through the lattice that was supposed to beautify the creepy darkness underneath the porch, the place where cats gave up the terrifying screams that accompanied their love. I am brought back to this childhood territory by the better side of the dirigibles' nature. Common earthly life was present in them (in many respects a body is just a body), but its form had been so transformed that it seemed they must have swallowed a potion, like Mr. Hyde with all his majestic lawlessness.

But their ability to work spells over us also can seem, at least in adulthood, like a degrading trick—the stack of porno magazines left beside the toilet at the fertility clinic, so insultingly unscientific. Now the flesh arrives daily, whenever

I dial in to check my vapor-mail, and it *is* like Mr. Hyde's, if he had set up a drive-thru franchise for his fizzy beverage. Relentlessly, this flesh scuttles after novel permutations, having exhausted the more conventional ones. But there are no novel permutations anymore, and I think of a line from John Berryman's *Dream Songs*: "We are using our own skins for wallpaper and we cannot win."

This is the primitive world we've re-created with our electronic wizardry. But way before humans arrived at any sophisticated ideas of commerce, sex in most animals made use of the economies of scale—lots of reproduction, lots of offspring produced with the slim hope that one might make it to adulthood. One of the most cherished books I own is my ninety-nine-cent 1976 copy of Haig H. Najarian's *Sex Lives of Animals Without Backbones*, replete with line drawings of protozoa blending and splitting. It contains also a sketch of the various copulating positions of squid. The breaching of various species of ovum, gametes moving like the harlequins of Cirque du Soleil. There is a drawing of hermaphroditic snails who pile orgiastically one on the other, penetrating whatever orifice is most proximate.

Professor Najarian doesn't come right out and state it, but his book is a testimony to the primordial birthright of our desires. We cannot help them, so we are innocents. He dedicates the volume to his mother.

With the combined forces of money and evolution and electronics at work, it seemed bound to happen that naked skin would exhaust itself. This exhaustion sends me back to my pathetic self, the self I have banished—and of course as soon as the mind banishes the actual body, then the actual body insists on barging into the Jacuzzi in the Hawaiian isles where one was attempting to build a modern-day diorama modeled after, say, something from a painting by Paul Gauguin.

There is also the problem of the wheelchair, which must be banished from the diorama, whereupon the wheelchair retaliates by barging into the scene too. One wants to camouflage it with garlands, or weeds like the ones soldiers in Vietnam wore on their heads, but that would only make it more obvious. I've thought of asking Jim to remove it, but doing so would make my faintheartedness too blatant. Instead let me look at it steadily and say, *Yes that is my wheelchair over there.* Oh no, that is too tough, so I close my eyes and enter a darkness where it wreaks havoc nonetheless.

From the first I heard of it, I was eager to see Pedro Almodóvar's movie *Talk to Her*, which builds its plot around the erotic potential in the afflicted body. The two female leads occupy slots far from the center of the spectrum of possible incapacitation—they're in comas. And the story makes use of doubles, two couples, two healthy men and two comatose women. One has been in a car accident when the movie commences, and the other, a bullfighter, gets gored while we watch. But it is the sight of the inert body being handled that makes the viewer squirm, as the male nurse, Benigno, rubs it with emollients. He opens her legs like the handles of a pliers so that he can perform the offices of the washrag and the menstrual pad. Her total pliancy is a parody of the pornographic ideal, and we soon grow confused over whether we are seeing acts of charitable love, or courtship, or duty, or perversion.

In the movie the women are, in a strange way, perfected. One good (if predictable) joke—when Benigno voices his intention to marry his Alicia—is that they will get along better than most married couples. The bullfighter's boyfriend, on the other hand, has a normal relation to his lover's comatose body, which means he is estranged from it and helpless in its presence. Hence Benigno's advice: *talk to her*.

Most of us tend to panic when confronted with the mystery of stricken flesh—we do not know how to fix it, and this is the cause of our estrangement and helplessness. There is also an iota of fear: of contagion, no matter how irrational, no matter how nontransmissible the sickness. As lovers *and* nurses, the men in the movie have a choice of only the perverse relationship or the inadequate one. This is a neat cinematic dichotomy, of course, about which we know one thing for sure: that the body's languishing will somehow be resolved in two hours, whereupon we will once again step out into the true and scary world that has no such finite starts and ends.

Scary because here the languishing can go on for years, and whatever allure the pliant body might have inevitably deteriorates as the caregiver is worn down by his duties. Almodóvar's movie does give to one of its women the cinematic cliché of the miracle cure, but coming to terms with my illness has forced me to give up on that possibility, which

I think caused the relationship between my psyche and my illness to remain childish, meaning that it was presided over by a child's false sense of immunity to time. While last year's therapist felt that my giving up on hope had darkened my outlook, I think hope shackled me to my body as it dropped like dead weight to the floor of the sea. And surrendering hope has left me feeling unburdened, lighter, strangely giddy as I float.

There is an erotic component to this surrender—it comes from the self relinquishing control, throwing itself away. Then the body is offered to whatever seizes possession of it—whether the seizer be disease or time or a human lover. Or it could be religious ecstasy—as in Bernini's sculpture *Saint Theresa and the Angel*, the saint's head tipped back with her eyes closed and her mouth hanging slack, again that half-bored, half-sleeping decoy face, signaling that the attention normally given to the world is being turned inward with all the intensity Theresa can muster.

I'm getting my picture of the sculpture from the cover of the book *Erotism*, by Georges Bataille, French philosopher of the sexual appetite whose thinking derives from a blend of Baudelaire and the Marquis de Sade. Bataille takes for his book's premise that *eroticism is assenting to life up to the point of death*. I don't know what this means in pragmatic terms, but my brain drifts in the same direction as the main current of his thought: that we are each so alone in our bodily organism-ness that our spiritual lives, and our sexual lives, act out our desire to achieve communion with something beyond the edges of our own skin. The egg and sperm's smashing together is the version of his thesis writ in miniature; in larger form, there is the example of the human falling down enraptured and speaking in tongues, an Esperanto that links the soul to a mystical race from the beyond.

There is also the larger drama that takes place in the bedroom, more serious than a game, sort of like the living tableaux that women would form at garden parties in the nineteenth century, the Three Graces with their limbs intertwined (I know about this only because I had to orchestrate just such a *tableau vivant* in my role as the mayor's wife, in our sixth-grade production of *The Music Man*).

You can see why these activities would be appealing to a cripple. Joining forces with someone else means a respite from fighting the body's ravages on one's own. Strife loves company, especially strife in which one is bound to go down the loser. Plus, it seems that if I can get deep enough into my body, maybe all its disturbing symptoms will disappear, the way the storm goes calm at the eye of it. And this *does* happen—a bit of good biology I chalk up to the pain-relievers called endorphins that are released by the brain.

There are also practical considerations: sex is usually accomplished lying down, a posture that camouflages frailty. Except, of course, now the bulge of the pump is always there.

To be partly human and partly a mechanical thing: this is a cyborg, in the parlance of science fiction. Sometimes the cyborg becomes an erotic object for her very freakishness: I have seen several *Star Trek* episodes that hinge on this premise. She has the stamina of the machine, plus the mystery of who-knows-what carnal apparatus. She has human beauty, usually manifested in a slightly abstract form, sheathed in silver skin or with a face partially occluded by a metal superstructure. Part of me thinks that being a freak is interesting—the great hunt of my youth was for some distinction that would render me more exotic than the run-of-the-mill other girls. And one of the most arousing memories of my recent life is Jim batting my hand away from where I was using it to anchor the hem of my T-shirt, this when the foreplay was just starting to take, him saying *I don't care if I see it.*

All my life, in health and out, I have hunted for communion—drugs, meditation, mountain-climbing, men, a variety of religions; I have sought dissolution of my physical walls, the body cast off like clothing stepped out of and kicked across the floor. Lately I've even looked at the maundering of that newest of Bataille's offspring, the art history professor in France who supposedly had sex under highway bridges with street people and stevedores. I understand why she would want to do it, though I see it a weakness in her character, this desire to cast off the body when there is nothing wrong with hers.

As far as poetry goes, the body in extremis has given us Crazy Jane and Baudelaire—or, for a more homegrown example, we could look at Raymond Carver's "Proposal," a poem that is partly about making love after his diagnosis of terminal cancer, surely a justifiable circumstance for self-relinquishment:

Back home we held on to each other and, without
embarrassment or caginess, let it all reach full meaning. This
was it, so any holding back had to be stupid, had to be
insane and meager. How many ever get to this: I thought
at the time.

How many ever get to this: see how the diseased want to be an ex-
clusive club, a mensa society of fornicators. We think our
love takes greater courage, no matter how limp our secret
handshake is.

And it occurs to me that someday I will eat these words
I've written here, because what I know most surely about my
erotic life is the fact that it is provisional. My body will have
changed by morning—and, in all likelihood, not for the better. And Cupid is a little guy whose energy seems liable to
flag as the body starts grinding through the hard work of
decay.

Because decay underlies it all, is both the substance of our
graves and the loamy below-porch catshit-littered birthplace
of the dirigibles (Yeats's Crazy Jane pops their balloonlike
forms when she says: "Love has pitched his mansion in /
The place of excrement"). I should also mention the second
of Bataille's great themes: how taboos arise in order that the
body's interior and exterior not be mixed. Blood and feces
are not permitted to present themselves in open air, except
under controlled and ritualized circumstances. Civilization
simply does not function when one loses control of one's
bowels in the big box store (this was not me, by some lucky
stroke, though I said to myself *You coward* when I did not

help the woman whose violating of the taboo I had witnessed in Costco; instead, I scuttled away like everyone else, afraid of how wildly, how flagrantly, she had swung an ax at the ice of my human heart).

Fear of the swampy wilderness in the body's interior is one of the idiosyncrasies of the human species. Wrote the diarist W. N. P. Barbellion in 1915, to show us how contrary the animal kingdom can be on the matter of this taboo:

> The vomits of some Owls are formed into shapely pellets, often of beautiful appearance, when composed of the glittering multi-coloured elytra of Beetles, etc. The common Eland is known to micturate [*note:* this means pee] on the tuft of hair on the crown of its head, and it does this habitually, when lying down, by bending its head around and down—apparently because of the aroma, perhaps of sexual importance during mating time, as it is a habit of the male alone.

Polite society imagines that the worst part of disability—the real horror of it—comes from how porous disease will make the corporal boundary, and as a result much energy goes into camouflaging the taboo's breakage. So I hide the bulky package of my disposable underwear underneath the bathroom sink. Once, when giving myself an injection of interferon, I hit a vein by accident and a rooster-tail of blood sprayed across the stark white kitchen. It was obscene but also thrilling, a phenomenon I was familiar with only because I'd read the novels of Denis Johnson. He sums up the taboo in one of the stories in his book, *Jesus' Son*: "There's so much goop inside of us, man . . . and it all wants to get out."

If examined calmly, I can see it's a needless waste of emotional voltage, the panic roused around the job of hiding the material leakage of the self. The Costco is full of shit, it will not be harmed by more; my dinner may spray from my mouth and my bladder may shudder around what it impounds, but it is still worth that uncontrollable raucous laughter when the right gang is assembled at the table. Jim has a quick wit and so he is especially familiar with all these leaks. The other day we were alone when my nose dripped on my lettuce leaf, and quickly I popped it back into my mouth for a joke—why can't the fluids return, they've only moved an inch, and they might have gone there in a back-sniffle anyway? *You're sick*, he pronounced—*ha! exactly!* It is easy for an invalid to get exhausted by the vigilance—that foremost among our mortal chores should be this job of keeping the goop inside.

When it comes to sex, though, what we want is leakage: for the essence of self to get through to somebody else somehow. And this applies not just to body but to mental essence as well. We want to experience the same ecstatic goop that's packed inside the person with whom we're trying to fuse. And we want that essence to be received not in words but in actual *feeling*, a direct body-to-body download—at least I do. I want my faulty neural circuits to be overridden and overwritten. I want some mental analogue of the copulatory experience of an eland.

The trouble is words, how they remain the barbed-wire fence wrapped around us that we can't climb: "If someone *says* to me what he has thought," writes the philosopher Wittgenstein, "has he really said: what he *thought*? Would not the actual mental event have to remain undescribed?—Was *it* not the secret thing,—of which I give another mere picture in speech?"

Sometimes I too turn into a philosopher when Jim and I go paddling on a river slow enough to leave us no real work to do, and on these afternoons deep in the shade of alder trees I will ask him: "Do I really know you? Do I really know what you *think*?" On this question, what Wittgenstein has to say is, "'Why does what is going on in him, in his mind, interest me at all, supposing that something is going on?' (The devil take what's going on inside him!)"

The question causes Jim also to turn into a crank: "You've known me for twenty years for god's sake! Of course you know me!" A man who favors action over deliberation, he thinks I invent inane speculations for the purpose of driving him crazy.

And to clarify Jim's position that started me off—*Nobody wants to read about you having sex*—I think what he meant was: *Why would you speak?* In answer, I can only say that a writer will sometimes deign to consider her audience, and it is my belief that people are generally interested in sex, probably even me having it.

Two-Man Boat

This morning is an odd, record-breakingly sultry one in June when the temperature has already topped ninety degrees. So we have driven a few miles, to the tip of the point that sticks into the southern end of Puget Sound. "Nothing is more dreary than a pleasure ground on work days," wrote the naturalist W. N. P. Barbellion in his journal (the first memoir about living with multiple sclerosis) in 1913. But today the harbor looks more surreal than dreary. Everything appears to be wrapped in plastic, like a sandwich.

To the north you can see the Olympic Mountains, dark blue ribbed with snow. We launch our boat here because the marina has a boat ramp. The boat, being inflatable, could easily be carried anywhere. But because I cannot walk, we need to get the truck close to the water.

The shore here is made of round stones pronged with barnacles. A stretch of muddy sand lies at the shore's lower reaches—visible at low tide, now. Straight ahead lies Dana Passage, where the current is strong, as we have learned from exhausting ourselves against it. But today we are going to turn left, into the large bay opening to the south, at the bottom of which, ten miles off, you can see the city's domed capitol and the port's loading cranes. The morning's heat has made the water glassy, in the chemical aspect of the word: it looks like melted rock, gray and dense.

The houses here are closely spaced, but when we clear the point the bluff grows steep and becomes unsuitable for development, and so it looks wild, overgrown with Oregon grape and madrona trees. With the annoying piety of those who choose self-propelled forms of travel, we curse the motorboats with their plumes of burnt oil trailing. There is nothing like a jet ski to wreck a fictitious wilderness. We are snobs, and the boat, barely more than a child's toy, is our high horse.

I have used up much of my life this way, in hours utterly without purpose. My embarkation goes like this: we back down the boat ramp, and Jim unloads the back of our old pickup. While I am reduced to waiting, I try to mitigate my uselessness by telling myself that my job is to observe. A blue heron swallows a fish by undulating its long throat. It regards us with disdain and walks a few steps off on its toy legs, shaggy feathers skirting the top of them like Josephine Baker's banana outfit.

In any chronicle of my kayaking, I have no choice but to include Jim, as I could not do this without him. The word *husband* seems wrong, with its suggestion that marriage confers some sort of virtue. But what are the other choices— "mate"? The robotic "other"? "Partner," with its law-firm connotations? Or "lover"—god help us. There is simply no good choice.

If I can manage it, I will have swiveled my legs so they dangle off the truck's bench seat by the time Jim sets up the boat. The heron flaps a few paces away, barely bothering to clear its feet above the shore. When Jim is ready, I grab him in a bear hug and he drags me down, my sneakers scraping across the ramp's concrete washboard ridges. It takes some finesse to drop my butt over the edge of the boat without tipping it. Once I am settled in the kayak, I am also set loose inside a pleasant fiction, that I am just like any other woman in a big hat, paddling.

Jim makes jokes when I ask him how my helplessness makes him feel, analysis striking him as ridiculous in situations that call for action. Instead, he offers whatever practical solution his own considerable strength can give, when faced with the disasters that have written the history of my body. He is like the person who lifts a car off a child, only in his case this is a phenomenon of daily living. Often spectators are alarmed when they see him dragging me. Then he becomes a hero when they learn what's going on. Once, in Hawaii, one of the ubiquitous beachside stoner-dudes applauded him for treating his mother with such tenderness.

And because we are pathetic, my knee-jerk reflex is to adopt one of a variety of (somewhat imperious) personas: the mute or curmudgeon, the hyena or duchess. In any of these personalities there is also an element of pride that I try to suppress—this paddling is harder for me than you, whoever you are. But the suppression of pride just feels like another form of it, the way beer carbonates itself by dint of being bottled.

This is the kind of payment I am expected to make on the debt my body has incurred: Jim wants me to participate in his rituals. He wants me to experience the ritual with him even at the cost of carrying me, and he wants my zest even if I have to fake it. Often I try to worm out of going, but I relent because I'm itchy to get out and see the day. Our kayaking is like sex in that emotional authenticity is not always a prerequisite, though it is supposed to be acquired by the time the activity comes to its conclusion.

Maybe a mile across the water in most directions lies another green mass: other harbors and headlands. This is no big open water; the sport is not heroic. All it requires is a high tolerance for boredom, for not much excitement beyond the occasional wake of a speedboat. Stories are made from one thing happening after another, suspense built from expectations that may or may not be satisfied, but rituals are made from repetition. And from the reassurance of the familiar, which is made holy as it is repeated.

Directly across sits Squaxin Island, uninhabited Indian land where a little state park used to operate, off-limits to the public now—though I did trespass there a few years ago when I could walk. On the island I took off my shirt and lay down on the rocks, and though Jim crabbed about my nudity we both did fall asleep, waking to the sound of footsteps, clack and clunk of rock on rock, and I remember thinking that if I kept my eyes closed I could stave off the inevitable encounter with the tribal police. But when I finally looked up, my eyes opened on the muzzle of a deer, chewing some grass and regarding my breasts. I even have a memory of the deer licking salt from the space between them, but I am pretty sure I've made this up.

The Indians native to this place traveled via canoes that were formed by hollowing great cedar logs and filling them with boiling water, wedging the hollow wider and wider as the wood softened up. Women's canoes were large and used for hauling cargo from place to place. They did the grunt-work of gathering, and the water floated the foodstuff home while they steered with their specifically sized women's paddles. So perhaps not exactly zest but gratitude is the proper frame of mind. Gratitude to the water that carried their tremendous burdens. And now, me.

Today we are going to a place we call Sand Dollar Beach. Because we're out in the open water where several inlets converge, there is a protected deposit of sand on the back side of a rocky outcrop. Some combination of currents keeps this cove free of mud, which would choke the dollars, clogging the little orifices that are their mouths, at the centers of their flat undersides. The water has little of the murk we normally travel through in town, down at the foot of the bay, whose surface is covered in the summertime with a variety of scums that I try not to blench when entering. It is a luxury to be sitting on top of this clear water. Normally, you can't see what dwells inside it unless there is a breach.

It's not uncommon, in season, to see salmon jumping, heart-jolting eruptions when the big fish breaks through and then whops down on the surface. I've been told this is how the females break up the ropes of eggs inside their bellies when it's time for them to spawn. Harbor seals also poke their heads out of the water as we go. When Jim echoes their huffing noises, they stretch their necks and rise to look at him, before eerily and silently sinking.

Inside the water, most visible are the jellyfish: white ghosts that propel themselves by fluffing. When they drift near the surface, I can make out what the field guide says are their gonads, especially distinct inside the large amorphous jellies whose center is occupied by an orange orb, like an egg yolk. At deeper than a foot, though, even the brightest creature is a blur. Whereas the hiker gets her crisp views in the thin air, the paddler gets mostly ominous portents. And this is not just paranoia—the egg-yolk jellyfish really do sting.

There are birds, of course, who traverse the boundary between water and air. And we who live on the air-side of that threshold tend to be spooked or stymied when we see the creature cross over, say if we see the grebe or cormorant submerge and disappear. We wait for it to come back up, but often it just disappears, refusing to give us a neat ending to the story. Because most birds head north to breed, just a few can be found on the water today, mostly the gulls and an occasional pigeon guillemot, a black seabird that arouses us in a way the gulls do not, when it flashes its glamorous red feet. But my gaze requires constant re-supplying; it digests the guillemot quickly and then moves on.

When I was a college student majoring in wildlife management, a professor once gave us the assignment of observing a bird for eight hours straight, following the same bird for as long as possible. I chose a blackbird and found the tedium unbearable—all it did was sit on a sequence of branches, occasionally giving its reedy tweet. Suddenly I knew I could never be a field biologist, a life marked by plodding most of all. My powers of attention were too deficient for me to ever be a romantic loner female biologist with an unkempt ponytail. What I imagine usually outweighs what I observe because life goes by me blurred.

The common run of us become inured even to the rarity if we are forced to sit with it long enough. I think of Robert Browning's poem "My Last Duchess" (see: in grad school I switched to being an English major), in which an odious duke dwells on his dead wife's portrait long enough to hint at his having had her killed. But then boredom sets in, and he skips on to some other idiotic rare gewgaw that he owns. And this is part of his offensiveness, that he cannot sustain his attention on anything.

I call this syndrome being "eagle-jaded," eagles having become common enough around here that they don't necessarily turn our heads anymore. Sometimes Jim and I will float by one perched on a piling, and the bird will outwait us, staring us down, until we eventually check our watches, then turn and paddle away. *How valuable am I?* it asks, and we answer: *Not worth an hour of our time, bub!* This is how it is with elusive creatures: we hunt them with fervor, and then when they appear, if they linger, we pronounce them not quite good enough.

I'm thinking about Emerson and Thoreau as I write this: the two craftsmen of our national mental template when it comes to both individualism and nature. "The great man is

he who in the midst of the crowd keeps with the independence of solitude," says Emerson in his famous screed, "Self-
reliance," which gives justification to just about any psychopath who feels he is possessed by genius. Thoreau, famous
for his solitary stay at Walden Pond (wherefrom he less-
famously frequently returned to his mother's house for cookies), similarly describes the kind of solitary life that is con-
tingent on good health. To either man, the kind of debt I'm
talking about—to someone else's body—would be unbearable, and it seems downright unpatriotic to live a life of such
lopsided physical dependency (in sixth grade I remember
learning the fact that Montezuma was carried from place to
place so that his feet would never touch the ground; it was
understood that his indolence marked his treachery).

But no writer of early America's vintage fetishizes the
body like Walt Whitman, whose *body electric* is a particularly
bad metaphor for someone like me, someone who is bar-
raged continuously by her nerves' stray volts. *If anything is sacred the human body is sacred. . . . And in man or woman a clean, strong,
firm-fibred body, is more beautiful than the most beautiful face.* In my
copy of *Leaves of Grass*, the poem that follows is devoted to
Whitman's ideal woman, or more exactly women plural, who
stand before him as embodiments of the *maternal mystery*.
"Now I will dismiss myself from impassive women," he
says—the kind of women he wants to rub shoulders with
are "tann'd in the face by shining suns and blowing winds":

> Their flesh has the old divine suppleness and strength,
> They know how to swim, row, ride, wrestle, shoot, run,
>   strike, retreat, advance, resist, defend themselves,

> They are ultimate in their own right—they are calm, clear,
> well-possessed of themselves.

If Whitman had been the breeding sort, his great-great-granddaughters would now be working on their belly-muscles at the gym.

The paradox of these three writers is how they all stand at a distance from the people they describe—like me, they are observers/imaginers, and though they celebrate humanity, they are never completely a part of it. Even the effusive Whitman admits into his poems no one on whom he was dependent, even though he became disabled by a stroke when he was only in his fifties.

Often I can't bear to let other people lift me, or even assist me with the simplest tasks—the gestures of reciprocal dependency that we'd make would veer into the territory of the lewd. Think, if you know it, of W. Eugene Smith's famous photograph of a mother bathing her daughter, deformed by mercury poisoning in Minimata, Japan. The familial bond dignifies the ritual and lends to it a privacy, whose lack—say, were they only nurse and patient—would turn the picture into one that could have been taken by Diane Arbus, interesting but grotesque.

I don't recognize the sand dollars right away when I see them down through the water. They look like purple crescents, their lower two-thirds buried—at first I mistake them for some kind of vegetation growing on the bottom. They lean from the current, all tilted at exactly the same angle. When it is living, the animal is covered with tiny spines and tube feet, which push tiny particles of food toward the mouth at its center. The velvety surface flashes as the tube feet wiggle when the animal is brought up to light. And the familiar white disk that we collect is just its skeleton.

Because the breezeless heat has sapped me, I want to be dragged into the water as soon as we land, where, in an inverse sort of tide pool exploration, I sit in the shallows waiting for whatever the water brings forth. Green kelp in wide rubbery strands. And a thicker warty strip mottled with a purple and brown camouflage pattern. Small shore crabs scuttle under the vegetation. My crab-crawl is of course not so nimble as theirs, as I hoist myself with my arms and scoot across the sand. This is slow going until Jim grabs my foot like a caveman and drags me out to sea.

Instead of truly swimming I often just float, a metaphor for much of my life, now that my body is a passive thing, almost inert. Such inertia, though, characterizes how a lot of life gets made inside this water: creatures release eggs or sperm, and depend on the current to mix them up. They load the numbers as best they can. Then the rest is luck.

Once Jim and I saw this process happening. At night, at a marine lab in the San Juan Islands, biologists had lowered a waterproof lantern into the edge of the sea. After about an hour, a foot-long pile worm entered the light's day-glo green aura: slightly phosphorescent, many legged, discharging clouds of sperm as it writhed. And soon after it swam away, the twice-bigger female came along, eggs brewing from her body in a viscous gel. The sight was majestic and awesome; we felt as though we'd seen not one but two dragons. The biologist snatched her up and threw her in a bucket.

But nothing so dramatic will happen today. If I weren't writing about my unseemly dependency, it would remain a private thing. And I suppose I should have mentioned the actual humongous dragon that is love, but such a beast would never fit in this small boat. Instead, I'll be its ballast, a soggy Lazarus being ferried home, after Jim lifts me from the water once again and hands me my paddle like a sword.

KNOWLEDGE GAME: *Birdsong*

All morning, from the laboratory of my bed, I've been listening to a bird. First a rising warble, then a flat buzzing
sound, ending in three notes of the same pitch—maybe
slightly descending? I can't tell. For almost fifty years, I've let
electric guitars sand down the edges of my brain, making it
hard for me to discern the subtleties of birdsong. I need a
stupid refrain to glue the tune in place.

The experts would tell me to try hearing the song as a
picture, this much I know—I don't know yet that there exists a whole history of such transcription, ranging from
standard musical notation to computer-assisted sonograms.
As a beginner at this game, the best I can do is write this in
the notebook on the nightstand:

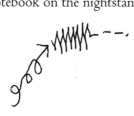

But these scribbles don't help later, when the pitch and timbre of the sounds have drifted up into the mental rafters.

It's a mystery to me, how the songs can be so *present* when the lips move over and over them. And yet how quickly they disappear.

When I finally get up and play the tape, the definitive tape made by the experts at Cornell, I hear nothing that matches my diagram. So this knowledge game is a game of loss. Songs imitated incessantly at 5 A.M. are gone by seven, in spite of my inscrutable graphs.

The problem with the definitive tape is that it contains all the birds in North America, with no efficient way to skip ahead to a particular bird that the field guide says might be present in this region. But sometimes I'll play the tape while I'm doing the dishes—this comes a little later in my pursuit of the knowledge game—and one song will call me to attention from my fog. Rewind the tape, and it's . . . *a Hutton's vireo*, though I'm suspicious of this identification because it sounds too esoteric for my woodlot. No, maybe not for my woodlot, too esoteric for me, inside whose brain the song is stored, below the brim of consciousness.

Nevertheless, the local guide says the bird is found here. Its song is a random string of rising squeals that become unrecognizable once I focus my attention on them (the way water held in the hand disappears when you lift it up to study). Perhaps the game works best when thinking is suspended and the ancient core of the brain is allowed to take charge.

The thinking me asks: *Is this game making you happy?* And the answer is: *No, no, you will never be happy. Best you can do is to fill yourself with the clutter of these distractions.* It's true that my nature usually feels the tug of gravity, that the fucking sunrise often makes me scream, what with the very idea of another day spent inside my fucking body. Sometimes the only thing that'll get me out of bed is my anticipation of the sensual pleasure of coffee, the most urgent of my desires. And I can do coffee at the same time as I can do birdsongs, outside— though I carry my cup in my crotch and sometimes it spills, which is the reason for the brown splotches on my shorts, in the region of my private parts.

It's not easy to be a bird-watcher when you can't walk. I have to bend my neck at an even more awkward angle than your standard birder to squint up into the trees. I do best with species that are willing to hang around, unmoving, at eye-level in the shrubs. Lucky for me, a few birds fit these parameters. But not many.

Hence the attraction of their songs, which penetrate space and in so doing bring the birds to me, even if I can't see them. All that is required is an open window, though on rare occasions I do coerce myself to leave the bed-lab and go outside at dawn, in the fleece costume that I've sewn to wrap around my tender shins.

The only thing I like about this picture, if I observe myself from outside myself (a daydream that's generally a mistake to entertain), is the black leather fingerless gloves I wear to push the chair, which put me in mind of Zorro. This part of my costume serves a practical purpose, though to be consoled by it—to *require* it for my consolation—seems childish. Childish to need some visible sign to direct at the neighbors, to counteract my stillness at this hour when I see them in motion, speeding off in their cars to zoom down the craw of another day.

I live on a hill that overlooks Puget Sound, its most-southern pocket, which is called Budd Bay. It's supposed to be the most toxic body of water in the state, though you can't tell from looking at its surface, which is always changing in accordance with the moon and sun. Its one constant aspect is its beauty—even though, to my ears, the word *beauty* sounds cornily outdated. We've entered the "post-beauty" era now, since we know how beauty can divert our attention to the left when on the right some atrocity is happening.

Here, to the south, to the right of the bay, spreads a wooded ravine. The luck of having landed in this place sometimes embarrasses me, especially when I think of the ragged people sleeping under their wet blankets on the shore. I assuage my guilt by telling myself that these circumstances are some kind of karmic payback—don't ask from what or whom—for my bad body-luck.

While the magnificence of this spot where I sit could only be improved by, say, an eagle swooping by (which happens from time to time), I'm also trapped here, because the road's too steep for me to climb under my own steam. The topography limits me—at times when I don't want to transfer to one of the motorized vehicles in my brigade—to a ten-by-ten-foot checkerboard of concrete and grass beside the driveway. This is my habitat now, bordered by a hazelnut tree whose fat leaves drape into the bird bath. A more patient woman could sit here until she'd trained the chickadees to eat right from her hand, and, while I like the idea of having such command over anything, I'm not sure this bird-taming would be conscionable from an environmental point of view.

In his book *The Snow Leopard*, Peter Matthiessen writes of encountering a crippled holy man: "Indicating his twisted legs without a trace of self-pity or bitterness, as if they belonged to all of us, he casts his arms wide to the sky and the snow mountains, the high sun and dancing sheep and cries: 'Of course I am happy here! It's wonderful! Especially when I have no choice!'" Whenever I feel claustrophobic in my grass-and-concrete checkerboard, I think about that holy man—how I should be more like him. But I also bet his cheery self-satisfactions would get irritating after a while.

My ravine contains a belt of maples that grew here after the old-growth cedars and firs were logged off years ago. The maples stand now eight stories tall, and they've become wrapped in English ivy, an invasive species, though we've snipped around the trees on our third-acre, so now their trunks are skirted with a wicker of dead stalks, which makes the trees look more in keeping with the post-beauty age. I call this place the Administrative Headquarters for the Empire of Crows, who I assumed were the birds waking up to emit not their normal *caw* but unforgettable screams that must accompany either murder or sex, though when I come more fully awake I never can remember the precise quality of the sound. It seems more suited to a word than a diagram, but I can't remember the word—huyyAEEE? nyeahungAWWW?

At first I blamed the crows, but now I'm beginning to suspect the Steller's jays, whose feathers on their black heads rise to one black spike pointing backward. I don't know for sure because I can't find those screams on the definitive tape, as if they were too horrible for the experts to include.

Though the ivy makes the habitat unnatural, my ravine is still a pretty wild place, especially considering that it's just a few feet from the driveway. So far none of my friends has been willing to go to the bottom because the ravine's walls drop off steeply, crisscrossed pick-up-stickwise by fallen trees covered in ivy. You set down your foot and find nothing there except a porous net of vines.

When I tell my friends, "Go down there as my emissary so you can report back to me," they tell me to forget it.

"Don't be afraid," I say. "I've heard there's old bottles in the bottom."

No—they might break a leg.

Then I glance off the cliff of my shoulder and say something like: "Well, I was the kind of person who'd go down there." That's the ground truth of me—hear how supercilious I sound? Not that I know for sure about the "supercilious," not that I can get to the bottom of myself and come back up with a verifiable object like a bottle, something I could hold for sure and study in my hand.

Ground-truthing is what biologists call entering an environment and actually surveying what is there via the senses of sight and sound. The advantage of sound is the way it pervades space— I don't need to be able to hike down into the ravine in order to hear what's inside it. Sound gives me not just a means for identifying the species that's singing, but in so doing it also provides access, giving me a way of entering the ravine.

Because I'm not yet initiated in even the most basic songs, for now I'm just taking notes—

1. (raspy intercom malfunction)

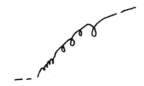

2. (operatic robot)

3. (melodic whip, like a noodle sucked)

Then comes the frustrating chain of processes—to consult the tape, to consult the book of local birds, before the memories of the songs evaporate. These consultations are frustrating because they seem artificial, so painstaking and unlike me, so dependent on technology and therefore one step removed from nature. Also, I've learned that the notion of a "definitive tape" is a fiction, because birdsong is more variable than the tape would lead you to believe. Since many birds learn their songs from each other, local dialects bend the tune just as they bend people's speech. There's a thousand miles of subtle mutations between a vireo here in the North-west and its song on the tape.

But eventually I gain a little ground—that raspy intercom (1) was a towhee, and the melodic robot (2) is song sparrow, at least I'm pretty certain, though the noodle remains un-known. (I found out later this was a Pacific-slope flycatcher. I'm not a good-enough birder to tell the flycatchers apart by sight, though I've learned that distinguishing their songs is easy because they remain fairly uniform from bird to bird. This is due to the fact that their songs are genetically "hard-wired" and not learned, as they are in other birds.)

While the unknown may compound the frustration, it's also what keeps this game moving along as one moves through incremental *aha!* moments enabled by the technol-ogy of books and the inaccurate-but-mildly-useful tape. Frustration is a prerequisite, a prickly sensation that goes away when you learn a song or two and start feeling a little smug—you've reached a plateau of complacency where you can take a breather.

That's when the game might be over, except pretty soon you hear something like a pennywhistle dropped into a fry-ing pan and you're back in the game again.

In the bird books, the songs easily parsed in English are writ-ten out that way. The chickadee says *Hey sweetie*, the olive-sided flycatcher says *I see you* or some other three-beat phrase (depending on your interpreter), but does my writing these phrases make it any easier for you-my-reader to hear the song? Probably not, unless you know the pitch and timbre of the words. Towhee is an onomatopoeic name, because the

that comes in raspy syllables is supposed to sound like *towhee*, although once it is cut loose from its moorings in the aural world and cast on a page passed from stranger to stranger, the word becomes merely a skeleton. Hearing the song is essential if the skeleton's to garner flesh.

Unfortunately, most bird songs can't find a good match in our crude human words. This results from the way the songs are produced, by a twin-chambered organ called a syrinx: two voice boxes working in tandem to produce music whose complicated polyphony requires a computer to catch all its details. *Syrinx* comes from the Greek word for panpipes, which seems appropriate—the bird's breath is driven through multiple chambers—and even sweet, lyrical at least. Until you trace it one step further back and learn that the word for panpipes comes from the reeds that a virgin girl let herself be transformed into rather than be raped.

To warn of danger: this is one reason why birds sing. But birds sing most robustly in the spring, when the males are gripped by the drive to mate and females submit to the most appealing singer. What appeals to me in birds' songs is the unabashedness of their desires, blasting so loudly I can almost forget my own body as I lie there listening while the sun climbs above the eastward mountains.

While driving around with Jim the other day, I heard a report on the radio about the ornithologist Don Kroodsma, who rides his bicycle across America each spring, zigging and zagging. His mission is simply to listen. I think he's trained himself into the mental state called synesthesia, a kind of neural cross-wiring in which the stimulation of one sense results in a perception from a different sense. A person who is a synesthete might, for example, taste mint as *a column made of glass*, though the most common form of these atypical perceptions is colored hearing. When Kroodsma hears birds, he sees a picture.

More precisely, he sees is a finely detailed oscilloscopic graph—a sonogram. He can hear a warbler in one county, then ride to the next county and be able to discern how that same species of warbler sings in a different dialect. He can also imitate the calls accurately enough to give the dialect's inflection. This man is a professor emeritus, the announcer says, which means he must qualify, by some measure, as old—and yet he sounds unwinded as he pedals.

I protest: "That's who I wanted to be. That's exactly what I wanted to do with my life." This is the kind of pronouncement I'll make after I watch, say, a figure-skating competition on TV. Suddenly I will want nothing more than to be a figure skater, always wanting to do the very thing I cannot do, even though I've hated skating ever since I broke my tooth on the flooded frozen tennis court at the village park when I was ten. At least three times a day I am overcome by such desires.

Jim says: "No it's not. You wanted to be a poet. You're doing exactly what you set out to do."

But of course I pictured myself as the poet pedaling her

bicycle across America, her legs shaped like stout branches of madrona.

This morning, outside in the checkerboard, I hear a song and flip through the pages of my notebook and am surprised to find a diagram that matches what I'm hearing:

The tape poses the hypothesis that this song comes from a ruby-crowned kinglet, a small elusive bird that I'm unlikely to see. Dimly I remember catching one in a mist net years ago when I worked for the Fish and Wildlife Service, holding it in my hand while I blew on its head to expose the hidden red patch. Its heart beat with a frightening force that seemed capable of tearing the bird's thin skin and making it explode in my hand.

Each bit of new knowledge in these knowledge games is supposed to serve the same purpose as the wads of clay and straw that pioneers once used to chink the gaps between the logs of their cabins. I chink the holes of my losses, like the loss of the mist net. The wind blowing hard is memory, and I'm trying to plug myself until I'm tight against it. Memory, okay, but without so much nostalgic attachment to my bipedal past.

In addition to these games, two general courses of action

would seem to be useful in the face of physical malfunction, one being the logistical solution, a solution like convening friends who would be strong enough—and willing enough—to carry me into the ravine (it's harder to come up with logistical solutions that allow for solitude). But my friend scolds me for even entertaining the idea of asking people to carry me into the ravine: "It's dangerous. You'd be asking them to get hurt. And what would you do down there anyway? You don't take advantage of what you've got right here." I hear her voice going *quack quack quack.*

I tell her I'd observe. "I'd sit down there for an hour."

"But you've never observed up here for an hour!"

"How do you know what I do," I sniff—a little nervous about her being right.

The other solution, the one my friend advocates, would be to quit wanting what I can't have—*cessation of desire.* Like the holy man, I ought to be happy with the driveway, the miraculous driveway, where a hermit thrush stands on top of one of the tomato cages in the raised bed. I know it's a hermit thrush because, and for the first time in my life, I can see the white whisker marks on both sides of its chin. This is the bird whose song Henry David Thoreau says "banishes all trivialness."

This bird is also about as close as we come in the New World to the famous nightingale that stars in John Keats's ode, and their songs share a similar downward-spiraling quality. Among the many well-known lines in "Ode to a Nightingale" is one that ends with the idea that "to think is to be full of sorrow" (echoing—rebutting?—Socrates' assertion that the unexamined life is not worth living). A year before the ode, he wrote an improvisation that sounds like a run-up to the more famous poem. It included the line: *O fret not after knowledge—I have none.*

This is the problem with the knowledge game. What with all my questing and all my fretting, it's hard for me to linger in the beauty of the song. John Keats does linger, and at first his listening sinks his mood, because mortality is what the song of the nightingale reminds him of, particularly the idea of a pain-free, easy death.

This would be a logical obsession for someone who'd just seen his brother die from tuberculosis, especially someone showing signs of the disease himself. In the painting made by his friend Severn, he's sitting in the woods at night while he writes the poem. Alarm is what registers most visibly in his white face, which is turned back over his shoulder toward the song, as if it scares him.

"Ode to a Nightingale" ends by addressing memory's inability to fix the song in place: *Fled is that music. Do I wake or sleep?* Evanescence, it seems, is a universal quality of birdsong. The expert on the bicycle is an anomaly. And maybe evanescence is a good thing because it forces the brooding to lift. It lets us forget that we ever thought of death.

When I was younger, Keats's high-flown language had no appeal, but now his central preoccupation is more urgent to me: How do we go on when the body's breakdown becomes impossible to ignore? The poem makes me remember that the world is full of things that should be paid attention to, even when they're darkened by the shadow of one's own mortality, perhaps especially when they fall inside that shadow. Life's meaning comes from the fierceness of this attention.

From a scientist's perspective, though, the contrast that Keats sets up—between unchanging birdsong (= the poem itself, the future famous words) and mortal man—is wrong. Birdsong changes: the expert on his bicycle finds a distinct lowering in pitch of the song of one species (the bellbird) in his thirty years of studying it. Nothing escapes transformation, and even the poem will change as its interpretation is ground by the years, as the New Critics are replaced by the postmodernists—and then the post-Beauty-ists, who see in every animal the putrefaction of its carcass and the decay of its song.

But in our small-run, temporary, and mortal-human days, we experience also the phenomenon of coming-into-being. Like: one early morning I hear a strange sound and write:

(whistle made of glass)

and by late morning, as usual, I can't fathom what I meant. But I see a cedar waxwing on the feeder and another one sitting on a branch in the ravine, and when I play the definitive tape, it turns out that the song of a cedar waxwing sings exactly:

(whistle made of glass)

A few days later I hear a song that sounds like a robin that's been hit on the head by a baseball bat (see: I've learned the robin's song, a hiccuping doodle I've overlooked all my life until this game turned my attention to it), and I see for the first time a black-headed grosbeak on the feeder, a bird that the bird book says sounds "like a drunken robin."

Then it starts to seem that by listening for their songs I'm *causing* birds to appear, that this game has the power to pull substance from the air, and I don't know why it ever made me sad. Delete the *fucking* from the sunrise, which is always beautiful, even when it's just the grayness lighting up again.

On the other hand: however irritable I am, I'm not insane. Do I really want to be outside in the damp when I could stay in the laboratory of the bed? Which is where Jim quizzes me as he prepares to leave the house at daybreak, "What's that?"

Flicker.

And that? *Steller's jay.*

That? *Willow flycatcher. Fitz-brew fitz-brew.*

Now, a Buddhist might argue that as soon as you jump to identify the sound, to give it a name, you've jumped away from the sound itself, and maybe this is the reason why the songs lapse from mind so easily—we rush from them too quickly. I've sustained my connection to nature by resorting to these games, yet I'm also aware of the paradox: that knowledge games take me out of nature.

And what about the beauty of the song itself, which I know I've overlooked in my quest for names? I'm not proud of the fact that I can't work myself into a state of exaltation when I hear the song of a hermit thrush, which sounds to me like *so squirrelly squirrelly*. It doesn't send me into raptures, but on the other hand, it doesn't fill me with woe, as it did Walt Whitman.

This year, I've learned the song. Maybe next year I'll be able to respond emotionally, once I know the name. Thought first, then feeling. *I think, therefore the winter wren.*

And to get a perfect score on Jim's quiz caused me to give my cackling one-ha laugh, because I know he expected to stump me. Desire again, the need to win, since it gives me pleasure—can't help it—to be in command of anything in the midst of my hermit-thrush-song-style spiraling down.

Jim sides with me when it comes to the ravine: he does not think that wanting to enter it means that I'm grasping desperately for what I can't have. He thinks that trying to come up with logistical solutions is a means of refusing to surrender. Desire is good; it leads us on. Our happiness should be greedy, should make us want more of it.

Then—action. Since my birthday approaches, he calls one of the Asian gardeners who advertise in the local paper, and Victor Hang (son of Huey, whose name is on the business card) shows up that day, a son with only the subtlest of accents, who seems a bit mystified about our project. But he says, well, sure, if we really want it, for six hundred dollars he can build a trail into the ravine. And though the job is scheduled for the next week, it's the next morning that a truck shows up, and not with Victor inside, who, come to think of it, seemed too well dressed for manual labor.

Instead he's sent Juan and Lionel, young Latino guys who attack the ivy with mattocks to unearth downed trees, which they rip with a chainsaw to make steps pegged into place with smaller branches. They find all the materials they need right there in the woods, no trip to the store, working so efficiently that the trail is finished by midafternoon. When Victor returns to claim his check, he speaks in his quiet voice from the bottom of the steps: "Ah, I see—at first I did not understand. But it is like Mount Rainier. All you need is a waterfall."

I'm studying his wife, a tiny silent beautiful woman who climbs up the trail in flip-flops until she's at my eye-level, smiling shyly.

By now the migratory birds like the grosbeaks and waxwings have left for their winter territories farther south, though a few species hang on, continuing to sing (if fitfully, now that their young have fledged).

My turn to descend comes a few days later, and I can't tell if Jim's lying when he claims that it's not hard to carry me down the path. All I'm required to do is not speak until we reach the muddy landing. He's bought a feeder on a pole and plants it: Happy Birthday. I am forty-seven today, older than I ever thought I'd be. My gift is the trail, the logistical solution, a nod to the refusal for it to be denied. The bottle at the bottom of the ravine turns out to be full of champagne.

We're sitting fifteen feet below the driveway, but we might as well be in the jungle—the nuthatches veer from our heads just an instant before they fly into our ears. How loudly we can hear the violence with which the air must be beaten in order to achieve the trick of flight. And the ivy is alive in a way I'd not noticed from up top, the leaves twitching and rustling, both from the birds hopping through their open slots and the raindrops that penetrate the canopy of maples.

We don't need binoculars to tell the difference between the three different types of wren, and I don't need the tape or a sonogram to tell me the difference between their songs because I can see perfectly well which birds are singing as they stand in the open with their heads tipped back and their beaks open. I imagine that the holy man's happiness doesn't hinge on this kind of attainment. He doesn't hanker after any infrastructure like this trail to take him anywhere other than where he already is, and he doesn't let fretting after knowledge interfere with his listening and the music's nameless seeping-in, as he sits in his spot in the Himalayas where the soil is too thin to allow for burial and the human dead are chopped up and left for the birds to eat.

To close that last paragraph, I was going to write "and then our bodies become the song," but this phrase, though melodic-sounding, is incorrect, I realized. The birds that take part in the "sky funeral" are vultures, birds that portion off the dead. And I can find no entry for vulture on the definitive tape, no song or call or chatter or whinny or drum. These graveyard-workers, the tidy-uppers of mortality, remain resolutely mute.

On Solitude

A tree falls in the forest without me to hear. This is an old riddle, almost a cliché.

Never mind whether or not it makes a sound, what I worry about from time to time these days is whether or not I care or, rather, about what form the caring should take now that the forest has spurned me, now that I can't enter it. Whether or not I'm bitter about that tree, the loss of the opportunity to hear its crack and crash.

Sometimes I do venture down a logging road, jiggling along. This sensation—motionless motion, uncomfortable under the ass and thighs—makes me realize that it wasn't so much the wilderness I loved as much as the feeling of my body moving through it, a feeling I loved best when my body hiked in solitude. The freedom of not having a companion whose speed I'd have to adjust myself to, whose pace would tell me, without words, whether I was fast or I was slow. Whether I'd succeeded in becoming what I'd hoped to be (a lone body conquering the wilderness—was that it? a body that transcended its gender?) or whether I had failed.

Solitude offers no gauge and no judgment. For the equanimity of solitude, I'd be willing to spend a day or week, whereabouts unknown, injured and waiting for rescue (my wilderness days preceded the invention of cell phones, and I'm glad about that; to have had such easy access to rescue would have shrunk the experience).

It used to pain me to live in sight of the mountains, as though I were living in a small town where I kept running into an ex-spouse at the grocery store, an ex-spouse who looked healthier than me and had already picked up a young lover, although after twenty years I think my rage/annoyance/grief has finally passed. In its wake, I waste time worrying about whether it's possible to tell the difference between "pure" memory—memory without sentiment—and nostalgia, a word derived from the Greek root for *home* and Latin root for *sickness*. Of course I am homesick for my former days. And yet we frown on nostalgia for smearing the past with a syrupy glaze. What is needed is another term that would allow us to long for the past with the accuracy of un-smudged recollection.

Or perhaps accuracy is incompatible with our reconstructions of the past, and our longing derives from their individuality, from the tilt we have given them. But don't some remembrances hold out the possibility of objective "truth"? Like the smell of the twenty bodies in the climbing shack, that male funk of sleep, and the groans like sobs that came with it? Or how I used my brassiere to wrap my friend's ankle when he twisted it at the top of Mount Rainier? Or the sound snow makes when stepped on at the summit, a crunch like the sound of burnt toast being bitten. Plus the sensation of the crystals underfoot, compacting into the waffle boot-print, grinding against each other as they settle?

No, not the bra—that was a different mountain. The rest I'm pretty sure I've got right though.

Now here I am. Back where my adulthood job-life started—at a national wildlife refuge. I chose this place for my destination because it's close enough to the interstate that my cell phone works, should the apparatus of my solitude break down (funny how I've come to welcome the idea of rescue). I wonder if people are happy to be paying for the upkeep of this kind of place, I mean a wildlife refuge kind of place, which is often not so picturesque and remains empty of human traffic; in fact, its purpose is better served without the human element.

Because the refuge lies only five miles from town, it does not have the desolate quality that many refuges have. It's mostly inaccessible meadowland, meant to be looked at through binoculars; no trails run though the center of it, so the animals can be left undisturbed. This flatland used to comprise a farm that stayed in business for sixty years until competition shut it down. Because of its location in the delta, the farm was not a viable business until a levee was built around it. Now people use the levee for a walking path, though boardwalks have already been built in preparation for the day when the levees will be broken so the meadow can revert to saltwater marsh. Then the mouth of the river will open wide again.

Levees and boardwalk: it's the kind of non-topography that's rare in the craggy Northwest. A place suitable for women pushing expensive baby-strollers that look like rickshaws. Its tameness offends me, though it's the kind of rollable wilderness where I can still be alone.

In his treatise about the two years he spent at Walden Pond, Thoreau wrote, "There can be no very black melancholy to him who lives in the midst of nature and has his sense still." No comment on what happens when sense abandons us; it's through bodily and mental health and strength, according to Thoreau, that we "come to know that we are never alone." Builder of cabins, sower of beans, Thoreau's body is the primary instrument he used in his experiment with living in relative isolation in nature. *Walden* is, at rock-bottom, the chronicle of Thoreau's body's trajectory through the woods.

When the legs become unreliable, one loses a large portion of the world. I get tired of the word *accessible*, the idea that the world must be reworked for my benefit. Instead, I start dreaming up machines that could take me anywhere; this technology seems easy when compared to, say, designing a little car that can be steered from 50 million miles across the solar system, over the terrain of Mars. A low-tech solution is for me to substitute companionship for solo travel, preferably the kind of companionship that won't impinge on solitude—which shouldn't be too hard since solitude is not a matter of being, in the strictest sense, alone. "The great man is he who in the midst of the crowd keeps with the independence of solitude," said Emerson, and *The Book of*

Famous Quotes contains plenty of this sort of advice, about how solitude should be a psychic space.

But the business of solitude has become troublesome for me of late. It seems natural for friends to draw away from my physical *unseemliness* as my body decays, and the plain fact is: I can't enter their homes anymore. Since I was never a social creature, this encroaching solitude might suit me, save for the fact that I haven't elected it, and the loss of choice in the matter grates against me. Of necessity, I've also begun to spend time in the company of people whom I pay to help me with the logistics of my living, and so solitude has become elusive at the same time as it's become oppressive, caught as I am in the push-pull of wanting more of it and yet resenting my involuntary isolation.

When I go to nature alone now, I have to work to squelch my fears. My mind clicks with the constant work of self-surveillance—Will I get stuck? Will I be forced to chew the bitter bark of having to shout for a stranger to help me? Today my nerves have already been twanged from driving here in the Rube Goldberg machine that is my old van—through a concatenation of wires and pulleys, the side door screeches open and a ramp lowers, on lucky days. Questions scroll across my mind: *Is this the last time I'll be doing this? Is this the end of my career as a solo traveler in the wild? What am I doing here anyway? Do I love this anymore?*

Too late for such questions: the van has arrived and the ramp operates successfully and I roll along the boardwalk that leads from the parking lot. I'm riding the kind of cart that must call up images of the elderly (though I try not to call them up), its basket loaded with the armamentarium of bird-watching. White snowberries hang on their stalks as the boardwalk *thock-thock-thock*s as I roll across the boards, a noise that doesn't faze a song sparrow who sits on a thorny purple blackberry cane, its few yellow leaves in the process of being mottled with smut before they fall. The bird only blinks with boredom as I thock past.

This refuge is located in the delta of the river that origi- nates from the Nisqually glacier, a steep corrugated tongue that lays off to one side of the route I climbed up Mount Rainier, what people call the standard or the tourist route (the word *tourist* uttered with contempt by the young men who worked each day on the upper reaches of the moun- tain). Climbing this route was easier than I expected and did not scare me, except when I had to step over a crevasse and snuck a glance into its bottomless blue hollow.

Probably my disease extended my life. Probably if I'd spent more time in the wilderness I would be dead already, being the kind of girl easily distracted, forgetful of correct procedure (in my grievance days I would have insisted on being called a woman, but *girl* seems more accurate, especially in regard to my ditziness). In the middle of trouble—the rock rolling down the glacier toward me, freezing my mouth in the shape of its *wow*—my mind flew elsewhere. Perhaps this was an early symptom of disease, this willingness to sur- render to whatever was about to happen. People prone to these states have no business climbing mountains.

When I worked at the park, I lived in a cabin by this river

ten miles downstream from the snout of the glacier, and for a while I sat on the bank each day and watched the little sticks that I threw into the river as a meditative exercise, to study the way they swirled. Usually they were swept downstream, but *slower than I expected*, and sometimes they entered an eddy that caused them to float uphill.

From these experiments I learned that the water does not offer what you want to see, and though the river is numbingly placid where its thick soup curls through the refuge, its currents are still dangerous. A few years back a man fell off a raft here—he'd paid to go on the land trust's fundraising trip—and he's never been found, however improbable this seems, since he was wearing a life vest. There are only a finite number of logs to get tangled under, and everything the river snags washes up eventually. Except those few objects that resist, as if they harbor a secret grudge against being reclaimed by a world where everything is categorized under its name and state of matter.

"Is that an ATV? Looks like a swell machine," says a fellow traveler of the boardwalk. These comments (of a sort I often hear) mean to show compassion, I know, though I'm taken aback by their illogic. I try to sound breezy instead of cranky when I say, "No it surely is not swell!"

But cranks are also hypocrites, and when it suits my interests I intrude on the solitude of others, like that of two hard-core birders absorbed in trying to identify some bird that sits on the ground, far off in the meadow, white with tawny markings. The birders keep quiet so as not to frighten it away—birders are usually the kind of people who seek solitude in the midst of their small groups. These two squint through the shrubs that border the levee, too focused on their bird to notice me.

"Harrier" pronounces a woman in a headband and glasses, the headband pulled down to give a scrunched aspect to her face, a near-replica of my own face with its glasses and ski cap.

"No, the head's not dark enough." This from her companion, an older man who seems to hold the position of authority.

"Some other raptor?" I suggest, feeling liberated by the fact that our interaction has no disability-angle to it.

"It doesn't have a raptor beak."

"How about a band-tailed pigeon?" I say, pointing to a tree. "A couple of months ago I saw a band-tailed pigeon in a tree right over there."

"Could be," he says without paying me much attention; he can tell I'm just a dilettante. Yet his *could be* makes me feel a little cocky, since I threw in the band-tailed pigeon from left field, not knowing what one of them really looks like. I like the way he ignores me, the respite from being noticed.

"Or a shorebird?" At this point I'm just casting about. "Too big."

"Could be a plover," the woman says in my defense.

"No, a shorebird wouldn't be alone this time of year."

"Mystery bird," concludes the woman, shrugging, as she lets her binoculars fall flat on her chest. When she asks me, "How about you? You see anything?" I take it for a victory— that momentarily I'm just another bird-watcher. And maybe not just a bird-watcher, but a true *birder*, despite all the hardware I'm encumbered with.

From Michel de Montaigne, we have this: *It is not enough to have gotten away from the crowd, it is not enough to move; we must get away from the gregarious instincts that are inside us.* I believed this sort of advice until I got sick, which is when I saw the benefits of cultivating gregarious instincts, a conniving and self-serving realization. I suddenly wanted—needed—to have a few friends willing to take me swimming at the lake, to push the wheelchair through the mud into water deep enough for me to float off.

I know I'm lucky to have such friends, even though their friendship is a paradox, because there in the black lake water, it's easy to do the kind of work that Thoreau recommends:

> By a conscious effort of the mind we can stand aloof from actions and their consequences; and all things, good and bad, go by us like a torrent. . . . However intense my experience, I am conscious of the presence and criticism of a part of me, which, as it were, is not a part of me, but a spectator, sharing no experience, but taking note of it; and that is no more I than it is you. When the play, it may be the tragedy, of life is over, the spectator goes his way. It was a kind of fiction, a work of the imagination only, so far as he was concerned. This doubleness may easily make us poor neighbors and friends sometimes.

The doubleness is what gives me pause—is it fair to call in my friends when they suit me, and then send them away when I'm tired of their company? Probably not, or at least I shouldn't pretend that I don't weave this hypocrisy into the increasingly complicated web of my human relations.

The trail ends at a decaying barn, a remnant of the dairy operation that's falling to ruin, its wooden shingles dropping and its white paint flaking off. The boardwalk ramps up to a viewing platform that's already occupied by a family—young mother, grandmother, three children, all in black windbreakers with a logo on the back of an aircraft carrier. Their loud voices pierce the air—the windbreaker family doesn't realize how hard I've worked to arrive here alone. If they knew, wouldn't they be using the hush-tones of church? Should I tell them to shut up? And if I do, will it increase the chances of this being the kind of momentous-enough experience that will adequately commemorate my last sojourn alone? Maybe then an eagle will fly over us, or maybe it will sit down on my shoulder. I'd prefer not to share my eagle with the windbreaker family.

But forget about the eagle; I have seen plenty in my life. Instead, we're looking at thousands of Canada geese who have settled on the meadow, fat brown lumps obscured by the fat brown clumps of grass. Today their honks sound high-pitched and *helpless*, rather than imperious, which I think of as their normal tone of speech. This vista from the viewing platform forces me to re-rig my definition of the wilderness, but that's all right—in former years Canada geese did nothing for me but annoy, what with their prolific bowel-expulsions and fondness for hissing at my knees. Now they're what I've been presented with, and not just a half-dozen expelling away down at the city park. Here, they're a thousand, or who knows how many thousands? Hard to tell, with the sun slanting low across the meadow's humps.

The windbreaker-women surprise me, and touch me, with their sensitivity for nature: they encourage the children to look out at the geese through the heavy spotting scopes that are mounted on the platform. I confess to having held the snobbish notion that they'd be more interested in shotguns and hounds, but instead the women are urging the children to study the geese, the sounds they make, the way they move. Everyone is vying for position at the scopes; the children and I use the one that's mounted low, while swallows loop from their mud-igloos under the old barn's eaves and carve figure-eights in the air.

These geese, I think, are the utmost Montaigne-ians and Thoreau-ites, finding solitude in the midst of their collective. Each is possessed with a dignified hostility directed mainly at plucking the grass. Their necks lunge as they forage, the whole flock engaged in the same motion while each bird remains utterly alone in its small rage. The force of the group housed in the fierce one, a forceful solitude housed in the fierce many.

You see their duality most clearly, though, in the choreography of their flight. Orchestrated by what collective mind or momentarily unified solitudes? Housed where, as they clap their wings in front of them, then rise and elect one of themselves to take the lead? Housed in a glance? Housed in the air, in a shift of wind?

Graciously, the windbreaker family leaves me in the dusk (*are you sure you're okay?*), so I can sit here and watch the geese fly off across the delta. Is this momentous enough, is this *sufficient*? From a distance, their groupings look like black ragged ropes constantly in the process of unraveling, setting loose a lone goose hoarsely honking. Then goose turns into geese again, as the rope rebraids.

From the Bardo Zone

Here in the country's top left corner, where there are only two seasons—rain and not-rain—the year's cyclical passage is punctuated by fish. Sure, there is summer, when the lawn's green blades turn into dry bristles, and there is also winter with its white peaks, the mountains revealed on those rare days when the sky breaks through the clouds. But mountains and blue skies are only the year's commas and hyphens, not the exclamation mark at the end of its paragraph. For that kind of rousing finale you need something on the order of a streambed full of dead fish.

For me, here's how it goes: come November I drive a few miles outside my small city, where a logging road zigzags through a clear-cut where elk sometimes wander. There's a brutal quality to the light that fills the clear-cut—it reveals the force of the human stamp on a place whose natural tendency would be to fill its empty spaces. But the road ends where the forest again closes in, around a clearing where squats a portable toilet's trademark plastic box. From here the trail heads into the mostly Douglas firs that border Kennedy Creek.

It's a location that falls pretty much in the middle of the spectrum of possible wildernesses. At one end of the spectrum might be a place like Seattle's Ballard Locks, where salmon move up a mazelike series of concrete steps, and visitors watch from a concrete bunker underground whose one wall is made of plate glass. When a fish swims by, viewers see it as if on a wide-screen TV. Proximity substitutes for the complete sensual picture. You can look into a salmon's nostril but you won't hear the thrash of the uphill fight. And you don't get the display of their extravagant deaths, which will take place later on the breeding grounds upstream.

Kennedy Creek is only a portable-toilet, five-miles-from-town kind of wilderness, but it doesn't hold back when it comes to the sensuality of death. As soon as I get out of the car, the first scent to hit me is that of fish oil mixed with the peculiar sweetness of rotting meat. The trail has been upgraded recently to a swath of black crushed rock, and there are signboards to fill in the salmon's backstory as well as to tell me how to comport myself. Do not wander from the trail. Keep your voice down. Apparently the water hears us just as we hear it.

What it sounds like is a washer swishing back and forth, the power cutting off then starting up again at a particularly explosive point in the laundry cycle. Less than a hundred yards from the parking lot there's a footbridge over a sub-thread of the creek, where many of the fishes' journeys terminate. Here, live chum salmon loiter in the company of the dead, which outnumber them two to one. This year the water level is high, and so the fish have traveled farther into the forest than I have ever seen them. The creek's tributaries plunge down the vegetated slope, and these notches are so steep and so scantly filled that it scarcely seems possible the fish could have ascended them. Such disbelief is the spectacle's human quotient.

Looking down from the bridge, I can see the living salmon mustering their resources in the creek's foot-deep pockets. Then they hurl themselves up on the gravel bars over which flows maybe only an inch of water. They propel themselves with their fins, their bodies wholly in the air, and not the slow wriggle one might expect but instead a spurt construed from brute force and will. Their shoulders—but of course they do not have shoulders—heave the rest of their bodies forward until they reach another pocket deep enough to swim in.

There's no hesitation once they decide to make a run for it. I see none who change their minds and give up, and head back, though often it seems their jaunts will leave them stranded. I watch a male battle his way upstream though I can see he'll be trapped by a stick that has fallen with one end in the water and one end on the bank. He noses at this solid wall that blocks his upstream passage. He swims in place with the undulating movements of a snake. After five minutes of dinking around in the crotch of the stick, he finally heaves himself over it, even though it rests halfway out of the water. Lucky for him, the effort frees him back into the main channel of the stream.

It's a lot to observe, these dramas in the creek, the many courtships transpiring amid the many dead. Fish hunker in the creek, a female and her would-be suitors quivering side by side. The dominant male will lunge over her back, weaving around her in a gymnastic pommel horse sort of foreplay, fending off any other male who attempts to intrude. She will have used a humping motion of her body to create a slight depression in the stones. Waiting beside her may also be other young males who've adopted the coloration of female fish, in the hope of sneaking under the radar of their bigger and more combative rivals. If everything goes according to plan, she'll drop her eggs and then a male will fertilize them with the cloudy substance of his milt.

Then death will set in, however contrary to Darwin it seems: this strange twining of procreation and mortality. Other species, like steelhead, do not always die after they breed, and so it seems there is an altruism inherent in the salmon's many deaths. They are animate tankers, ferrying particles from the ocean to this semi-urban forest. Traces of their carcasses have shown up in 137 other vertebrate species. The world is made of dead stuff, anyone who's walked in the fallen leaves knows that. But animals we feel compelled to bury, if they enter the visual field of us humans who admit into our presence so few reminders of our own susceptibility to the state of being dead.

The spent fish twirl in the water, whitening. It is hard to tell if they are breathing, or if the gills' movement is just a flutter caused by the current. The fish who die in the water tend to lose their skin like scarves, and then the flesh similarly peels off. The carcasses that have somehow ended up on land (has the water level dropped? or was the carcass dragged by an animal?) often lie curled in a crescent, the dry fins brittle as potato chips.

The trail drops down a clay bank and ends at the edge of the main channel of the creek, a clear and shallow laminar flow moving over the round stones. The water level's being so high masks the presence of the fish, but I can see their backs intermittently breaking through the surface at the margins of the creek. Someone has left a female and a male carcass here for contrast, the trail's final instructive tableau. In the water, a chum salmon's sides are brightly marked with purple streaks that resemble bruises. Dry, though, their colors are less remarkable than their forms. The male has a large hump on his back, a more aggressive mien. Not that the female doesn't have more than an adequate number of sharp teeth. But the male's jaws are outsized, a transformation that took place as he swam up here, as his body readied itself for breeding's violent work.

However, these two fish, left nose to nose, are not what most snags my attention. On the far bank there's a stump broken off a good four feet from the ground. And balanced on top, with its rigid body curled, there's a salmon. So of course I start to wondering how it came to be there—a drop in the water level, an itinerant bear? Or could it have fallen from the talons of an eagle, could so random of an accident have brought the fish to land so precisely on a ragged stump?

No, I decide, no accidents here, everything is scripted— the salmon governed by memories and maps that are somehow coded in their neural circuits. As the crow flies, we are not so far from the ocean. But to travel there by water would mean swimming past a dozen cities. And a dozen dozen watersheds, each cataclysmically altered by the twentieth century. In this ravaged waterscape, a fish must find its way to the ocean and then find its way back. The very complexity of such a system conspires against its continuance in an age that favors the monocultural crop, the half-hour sitcom, the drive-thru burger joint, the big-volume discount store.

So no, no accidents here, and the salmon perched high on a stump seems to have been put there to take our intellects down a peg. After half a century of study, we still don't know how they navigate to and from the sea, and it humbles us because, if there's one thing we do know, it is that if we lived in their shoes—okay, their fins—we could not replicate this feat.

In photographs taken by Scott Chambers, a former commercial fisherman whose body has been transformed by the neurological disease that used to be called St. Vitus' dance, the mostly dead salmon look up at us with eyes that seem to be made out of bright foil. These are humpback salmon, also called pinks, also called rags because of their comparatively mushy flesh. Solidity is not one of their bodies' defining traits, and often in the photographs the fish's body appears to be half-fused with the rushing water.

Chambers has named these photographs the Bardo series, from *Bardo Thodol*, which is the Tibetan title of what English speakers have traditionally called *The Tibetan Book of the Dead*. A more accurate translation is what scholar Robert Thurman makes the subtitle of his version: *the book of natural liberation through understanding the in-between*. It's not death that is the book's true subject, but that amorphous estuary that is no longer life and not yet death.

So *bardo*: the in-between, the zone between two states of form. Thurman identifies not just the bardo between life and death but also a half-dozen other bardos we move through as we pass from waking to sleep to dream and back. Our lives are a sequence of transitional states that we fuse into a fluid whole.

In the Western tradition we get concurrence from Heraclitus, one of the earliest Greek philosophers, who wrote:

> As souls change into water
> on their way through death,
> so water changes into earth.
> And as water springs from earth,
> so from water does the soul.

Heraclitus saw the nature of reality as flux. His famous aphorism, about our never being able to step into the same river twice, goes on to say that *so I am as I am not*. If reality is flux, then it follows that we live in a constant state of bardo.

One of Chambers's photographs translates this betweenness into the literal language of bones and flesh. A dead fish lies on the gravel, the rear half of its skin shrugged loose like a garment, from which the spine extrudes in a compressed arc until it joins up with the head. The purging of the flesh is incomplete, though; only half of the bones have achieved that state of incandescent whiteness that emerges in the late stage of its rot. For now, the fish is something for which we do not have a name, something in between a carcass and a skeleton. And the namelessness sits awkwardly on us who are used to having things one way or the other: you're a man or a woman, you drive to work on one side of the road and drive home on the other. You can see why the system has its advantages. There's a survival value in avoiding the head-on crash.

With my human mind I can't help speculating about what transpires in the minds of those who lie immobile, languishing, their color drained but the gills still moving. However foolish this mental exercise may be, it seems likely the fish have some form of understanding that their bodies are no longer functioning as they once did, an understanding that the neuroscientist Antonio Damasio might categorize not as consciousness but as emotion. Damasio offers the example of the marine snail *Aplysia* to support his contention that even a primitive creature will give some bodily indication of an emotion such as fear. Touch the snail's gill and its heart rate shoots up, ink will shoot out. The snail may not be able to do the processing of these emotions (which is what would turn emotion into something more akin with human feeling), but their presence is necessary to guide the actions the creature will need to make in order to survive. It's emotion, claims Damasio, that enables us to read our environment and keep ourselves alive.

So I wonder how the living salmon read the water in

which float the corpses of their comrades. They must have a perception of at least the basic physical properties of their immediate environment, the depletion of oxygen caused by so much decaying matter. And surely the spawned-out fish experiences a host of symptoms like lassitude, dysfunction, maybe pain. I don't believe they "think" about these symptoms, but some registering of them must be present, as this recognition is, after all, what enabled the fish to survive its younger days in a series of complex environments.

Damasio calls consciousness, conscience, spirit, and soul "one big region of strangeness" that sets humans apart from other animals, and what has in theory been our monopoly on these theological-ethical-cognitive zones also has given us a sense of entitlement in our governance of other creatures. Hence our right to eat them, to manipulate their habitats, to use them in experiments that will, with any luck, lead to cures for our diseases. And believe me, I do want those cures. But it is hard to look into one of the bright foil eyes of the Bardo photographs and then believe that soul and spirit are strangenesses to which only the human species can lay claim.

In another of Chambers's photographs we see what looks like an organized phalanx of fish, more than a dozen moving as a regiment against a substrate of leaves. But something about the fish's coloration is not right, their backs pale and their undersurfaces darker, and then you realize that their dorsal fins are not dorsal fins at all—instead it's the pectoral fins, the ones near the gills, that are breaking through the water. The fish are floating upside down, barrel-rolled by the air bladders in their stomach cavities.

There is something frightening about them, frightening because they are beyond our reach. Biologists speak of "managing" a living resource, intervening in the natural history of a creature to make it more compatible with human life. But this army of dead salmon is not listening to us anymore. It's as if death has inoculated them against our interventions.

In her poem number 1691, Emily Dickinson coins her own word for the dead's ungovernable nature:

> The overtakelessness of those
> Who have accomplished death
> Majestic is to me beyond
> The majesties of Earth.
>
> The soul her "Not at Home"
> Inscribes upon the flesh—
> And takes her fair aerial gait
> Beyond the hope of touch.

Here, as in the *Book of the In-between*, death is work to be "accomplished," and those who have succeeded in this work can no longer be overtaken by us who remain locked in our gravity-bound flesh. In Dickinson's version of death's conversions of the body, the soul then gambols off into the sky—and it is curious how many paintings of spawned-out salmon show them inhabiting the medium of air, as though they no longer float in the water because they have become substances made of breath.

"Ghost salmon" one might say, just as, looking at spawned-out fish in the real world of the real wild, they do seem to glow with the spectral quality of ghosts. In the cases of some dead fish, this analogy makes visual sense, as they are often covered with a white fungus that resembles snow. In one of the Bardo photographs the fungal fish hangs in a riffle of whitewater, its pose a mimic of that with which it fought its way upstream.

In his book *Totem Salmon*, Freeman House, another former commercial fisherman, sees the metaphor of the ghost playing out in the salmon's natural history, not just in the individual fish but also in the salmon population as a whole. House reminds us of the pains that we call phantoms when they inhabit the missing limbs of amputees, evidence of the nervous system's remembrance of the part that has been lost. Likewise, the environment "remembers" those species that have been cut from it. "The local field of being that we call the ecosystem," theorizes House,

> must experience a period of adjustment when one of its organisms has disappeared—even if the disappearance has occurred over a period of time beyond human understanding. When people, accidentally or purposefully, experience engagement with these fields of being, the direct, ineffable sense of the ghosts of lost creatures may come visiting.

> The ghosts are globes of emptiness floating through the bloodstream of life, nearly lost memories of the void left by some absent life form. Ecosystem absences can become palpable presence, a weird stillness moving against the winds of existence and leaving a waveform of perturbation behind. Most humans are slower to see and feel in this realm, sur-

rounded as we are by the noise of machinery, the buzz and hum of electricity. We need a tsunami of absence to get our attention.

I think this interpretation of the depleted world wouldn't be lost on the Tibetans, in whose scheme of things—as we are born and die and are born and die again—we ping-pong between realms that include humans, animals, and ghosts (and also hells and demigods and gods). It is easy to conceive of a Buddhist ether where globes of emptiness float around waiting to be filled by consciousnesses whose body-vessels have run their course. We snag a globe on the fly and are born into our next life, and the *Bardo Thodol* is a how-to manual on navigating what it calls "the terrors" that will face us between lives.

What the book contains is a series of prayers to be read to the person who has knocked on death's door and now waits for death to answer. Though one of the book's operative words is *compassion*, it also insists above all that the task of death be approached with a clear head. In Robert Thurman's translation, the prayers have all the briskness of a boot-camp drill:

> Hey! Now when the life between dawns upon me.
> I will abandon laziness, as life has no more time. . . .
> This once that I've obtained the human body
> is not the time to stay on the path of distractions.

Elsewhere the imperatives are even more forthright, reminding me of nothing so much as that point in old movies when a character is momentarily overtaken by hysteria, and the hero with a cooler head has to slap the hysteric's cheeks.

"Hey Noble One! Listen Without Wavering!" is the common opener to the prayers, which are to be read to the one who traverses the landscape of the in-between so that his/her mind doesn't run the risk of "riding the horse of breath like a feather blown on the wind, spinning and fluttering."

In truth, I don't know if I could handle having the *Book of the In-between* read to me if I were dying. The hierarchy of its afterlife seems another order of magnitude more complicated than life itself, and life itself possesses a degree of complexity that I barely feel equipped to negotiate. And then there is also the frightening aspect of its metaphysics, with fierce deities such as Yama, the naked hard-on'd blue-black fire-breathing-buffalo-riding god of the underworld. But one of its more reassuring aspects is how it puts the dying mind in the driver's seat. *Be fiercely courageous!* is my favorite of its exhortations.

Salmon are so totemically identified with the Northwest that viewing their runs is one of the inaugurating rites for new citizens of the region. Another rite might involve buying whole fish cheaply at the Indian reservation's tent stand and grilling them on the barbecue. There are seven indigenous *Oncorhynchus* species here, and most of them have several names—so another rite of immigration is mastering the lingo: coho sockeye humpy chum. And is it just a coincidence that this happens to be a near-homonym for the chant that is a Buddhist mainstay? *Om mani padme hum*, which Thurman says means "all is well with the universe, the force of good and love is everywhere and competent to help all beings out of every difficulty." A nice idea, though I don't know if I buy it. Stubbornly I cling to the material realm: *coho sockeye humpy chum!*

Yet eating salmon is a morally troubling act, because the fishing industry has hurt so many of their populations. And a person doesn't even have to eat salmon to be a destructive force. The houses we live in are made from trees that once shaded salmon streams, and the dead limbs of those trees once kept carcasses from being swept downstream. The forest that's been cleared to accommodate us once prevented dirt from muddying those streams. The electricity it takes to run the laptop that I write this on comes from dams that block their migratory routes; the runoff from the roads we drive on are full of toxic gook. The very act of moving here was probably the worst turn I ever did for the fish, as their numbers have dropped in inverse proportion to the burgeoning of the region's human population.

I originally came to the Northwest to work as a park ranger, but after one particularly arduous summer I noticed that something strange was happening to me. I had no diagnosis, and yet I knew my body was changing—its muscles had become unreliable, as if they were no longer fully solid. My arm would sometimes act like an arcade crane that has trouble grabbing even the lightest toy. And my legs turned rubbery, or a jolt of electricity would sometimes travel down their lengths.

That was twenty years ago. A couple of months later the doctor showed me pictures of my brain dotted with white spots, which glowed as brightly on the magnetic-resonance images as the fungus on a fish. And though my acquisition of debilities has been slow, it has seemed as though I inhabited a liminal region that was a twilit version of "normal" living. But maybe this is a form of self-aggrandizement, seeing oneself as a walking (or not walking) member of the dead.

Now when I go out to Kennedy Creek, I ride the trail on an electric scooter. I am glad for the chance to let my physical self dissolve into the wind and the trees, but other human spectators keep reminding me that the trees are *they* and I am *me*, a hunk of meat with no stamina for the wilderness.

Don't get me wrong; I'm grateful for the people who push me out when I bog down in the mud. But it drives me crazy when someone tries to take me aside (that is, if you can take someone on a motorized vehicle aside) to say: *I think it's great someone like you is out here.* Someone like me, meaning not like them, and thus do I get corroboration, in my aggrandizement, about inhabiting the bardo zone. Meanwhile, the gulls squawk from the trees: *the scrap! the scrap!* They too do not belong here in the canopied forest. Giving me the hairy eyeball, as if they want to strip a tendon off of me.

Scientists don't really know how salmon navigate: the smell of the birth-stream appears to be crucial, but olfactory recognition would not explain how salmon operate once they get out of sniffing range. I think of our not-knowing as another sort of bardo zone, in that not-knowing forces us to abandon categories and slots as we hover between hypotheses. Freeman House grapples with the mystery of salmon by concluding that the best way to study it is by means of contemplation:

Reductionist science attempts to understand the lives of salmon in separation from their field of being, the living sea. And we don't have the intellectual or perceptual tools to consider the interactions in a milieu so different from our own. . . .

If our engagement with natural processes is beyond our ability to measure and quantify in the laboratory, it may be that the only way to immerse ourselves in those processes is through the long practice of cumulative attentiveness. In the close-mouthed world of reciprocal perception, there is no way to learn to live in place but from the place itself. Even the waters can teach us, if we can quiet our appetite for "rational" explanation.

In lieu of this kind of quiet, most of us attempt to come to terms with the mind of the salmon by metaphorizing their navigational abilities in terms of our own way-finding inventions. But of course salmon don't have compasses or maps, only the mysterious receptor that is their body, which is able to measure, in the words of House, "the buzz and pulse of electromagnetic fields and currents, infinitesimally minute differences in temperature and salinity and light and food." Some day we may figure out how the body registers these properties, but the mind that processes this information will likely remain elusive.

Chuang Tzu, the Taoist poet from sometime around the third century B.C., made man's interaction with the natural world his chief subject of study. His poem "The Joy of Fishes" comprises a dialectic on the subject of man's attributing human emotions to animals. In Thomas Merton's translation, it begins:

> Chuang Tzu and Hui Tzu
> Were crossing Hao river
> by the dam.
>
> Chuang said:
> "See how free
> The fishes leap and dart:
> That is their happiness."

A conversation ensues about how Chuang can know whether or not the fish are happy, and the poem ends with Chuang winning the debate by insisting on Hui's precision of speech:

> "What you asked me was
> *'How do you know*
> what makes fishes happy?'
> From the terms of your question
> You evidently know I know
> What makes fishes happy.
>
> "I know the joy of fishes
> In the river
> Through my own joy, as I go walking
> Along the same river."

What I like about this poem is how it tells us that it's okay to cut ourselves some slack when it comes to our habit of anthropomorphism. When it comes to other minds, the best we can do is imagine an analogue of our own mind, and Chuang Tzu is suggesting that it should be obvious that when we make a statement about the minds of animals we are really talking about ourselves.

What is obvious about the people who come to Kennedy Creek is that they too are seized by joy. No mere sign can keep the children from squealing, and even adult visitors are liable to give out cries that have been forged by their amazement. Fleetingly, I get the sense we should not be here, trampling the bank and transforming the woods into a sort of piscine theme park. But staying home would be another form of betrayal, because it would be too easy then to forget about the fish and how their population is faring. And it is also good that we be reminded that the stink and decay we generally find abhorrent also has its place.

By now the Northwest has seen more than a decade of legal wrangling over whether twenty-six populations of salmon should be on the federal list of species that are threatened or endangered. At issue is the distinction between wild fish and those reared in hatcheries, which have churned out salmon in this country since the late nineteenth century. Such was the industrial era's faith in technology that its fixes, such as hatcheries, were seen as perfectly adequate substitutions for wild systems that evolved over the course of a hundred thousand years.

Of course each technological fix usually breeds new glitches, such as the various behaviors of hatchery fish (like reduced fear of predators) that leave them vulnerable to living in the wild. And so it would seem crucial to the species' long-term survival to preserve the genetic diversity of wild fish, although populations of some of these wild runs have dwindled to less than a hundred fish. Already so much inter-breeding has taken place that, genetically, salmon inhabit a bardo zone, a state of being neither this nor that, neither fully hatchery-produced nor fully wild, a threshold from which biologists hope to coax them back by building up wild populations.

The natural world has a way of backlashing when tech-nology attempts to meddle, and the environmental move-ment of the past century was founded on cases where the in-dustrial world's blind faith in itself caused the balance of nature to go awry. And because scorning technology was one of the poses of my young adulthood, it is ironic and painful to me that I find myself so completely lashed to the man-made world. Now my presence at Kennedy Creek requires a hundred pounds of plastic and metal and toxic chemicals, a battery-powered juggernaut that can roll only across terrain that has been cleared. I know I am only one small woman trammeling the wilderness. Still, it grieves me that I do trammel. What I would embrace, I crush.

I'm also not sure how I feel about the whole idea of karma. On the one hand, it makes me sort of edgy to think that my body's hard luck might be due to the fact that in some for-mer life I was a major bitch. And I fear that in this life I have been so weak-willed and lazy that I might be reduced to the realm of the hungry ghosts in the next.

It is almost spooky: how salmon put the *Bardo Thodol*'s reincarnation hypothesis into physical form. The dead one's molecules scatter, to become maybe part of those 137 other species. That is both thrilling and hopeful to me, the idea that someday some molecule of me could be incorporated into the agile body of a coyote. Or something not even so glamorous, like a long-tailed weasel. Or a Cope's giant salamander. Or a glaucous-winged gull.

Western culture finds a sign of its sophistication in the extent to which the human body is removed, via chemical means, like the pharaohs, from rot's cycling of molecules—no longer are we allowed to simply become food (well, we have made ourselves a slower meal for tinier creatures). Public hygiene dictates that our bodies not be left on scaffolds or chopped up and fed to carnivorous birds. And we have cultivated our primal taboos about the dead body at the same time as medicine has come to occupy a quasi-spiritual place in American life. The combination of these forces has led many people to view death as an aberration that we'll soon be able to conquer through science and the proper frame of mind.

Yet our unsuccessful hunt for other life in the galaxy tells us that life itself is the aberration, a quirky miracle we've been allowed to participate in—which for some is proof enough of God and for others is what makes antidepressants superfluous. Still, death is our default mode, and the process of maturation means coming to accept our mortal nature with humility and wonder. And the salmon—in their one and their many—ask/s us if we get this.

SOURCES

Aeschylus. *Prometheus Bound.* Trans. Philip Vellacott. New York: Penguin, 1961.

Aristophanes. *The Birds.* www.gutenberg.net.

Barbellion, W. N. P. *The Journal of a Disappointed Man.* 1919. Pocket Classics. London: Alan Sutton Publishing, 1984.

Bauby, Jean-Dominique. *The Diving Bell and the Butterfly.* New York: Knopf, 1997.

Baudelaire, Charles. *Les Fleurs du Mal.* Trans. Richard Howard. Boston: David R. Godine, 1982.

Brodsky, Joseph. "An Immodest Proposal." *New Republic.* November 11, 1991.

Burton, Robert. *Anatomy of Melancholy.*

Cederholm, Jeff, et al. *Pacific Salmon and Wildlife: Special Edition Technical Report.* Wildlife-Habitat Relationships in Oregon and Washington, 2000.

Chuang Tzu. *The Way of Chuang Tzu.* Trans. Thomas Merton. New York: New Directions, 1965.

Clark, Ella. *Indian Legends of the Northwest.* Berkeley: University of California Press, 1953.

Collins, Billy. "Purity." In *Sailing Alone Around the Room.* New York: Random House, 2001.

Cornell Laboratory of Ornithology. *Western Bird Songs*. Boston: Houghton Mifflin, 1992.

Cruickshank, A. D., and H. G. Cruickshank. *1001 Questions Answered about Birds*. New York: Dover, 1958.

Damasio, Antonio. *The Feeling of What Happens*. New York: Harcourt Brace, 1999.

Dickinson, Emily. *The Complete Poems of Emily Dickinson*. Ed. Thomas H. Johnson. Boston: Little, Brown, 1960.

Eagleton, Terry. *Sweet Violence: The Idea of the Tragic*. London: Blackwell, 2003.

Emerson, Ralph Waldo. *Essays: First and Second Series*. Intro. Douglas Crase. New York: Library of America, 1990.

Glück, Louise. *Proofs and Theories*. New York: Ecco Press, 1994.

Griggs, Jack. *All the Birds of North America*. New York: HarperPerennial, 1997.

Heraclitus. *Fragments: The Collected Wisdom of Heraclitus*. Ed. Brooks Haxton. New York: Viking, 2001.

Holt, Jim. "The Human Factor: Should the Government Put a Price on Your Life?" *New York Times*, March 28, 2004.

House, Freeman. *Totem Salmon*. Boston: Beacon Press, 1999.

Hyde, Lewis. *The Gift: Imagination and the Erotic Life of Property*. New York: Vintage, 1979.

Introduction to Aristotle. Ed. Richard McKeon. New York: Modern Library/Random House, 1947.

Kael, Pauline. *5001 Nights at the Movies*. New York: Holt Rinehart and Winston, 1982.

Kaplan, Justin. *Walt Whitman: A Life*. New York: Simon & Schuster, 1980.

Keats, John. "Ode to a Nightingale" and "Ode on a Grecian Urn." In *The Norton Anthology of Poetry*. 4th ed. Ed. Mary Ferguson, Mary Jo Salter, and John Stallworthy. New York: W. W. Norton, 1996.

Kroodsma, Donald. *The Singing Life of Birds: The Art and Science of Listening to Birdsong*. Boston: Houghton Mifflin, 2005.

Lemmon, Robert. *Our Amazing Birds: Little Known Facts about Their Private Lives*. New York: Doubleday, 1951.

Martin, Laura. *The Folklore of Birds*. Old Saybrook, Conn.: Globe Pequot Press, 1993.

Mitchell, Stephen, trans. *The Book of Job*. New York: Harper-Perennial, 1979.

Montaigne, Michel de. *The Complete Essays of Montaigne*. Trans. Donald M. Frame. Stanford, Calif.: Stanford University Press, 1957.

Moore, Marianne. "An Octopus." In *Modern American Poets: Their Voices and Visions*. Ed. Robert DiYanni. 2nd ed. New York: McGraw-Hill, 1994.

Motion, Andrew. *Keats*. New York: Farrar, Straus & Giroux, 1998.

Nagel, Thomas. "What Is It Like to Be a Bat?" *Philosophical Review* 83.4 (1974): 435–50.

"Nutria in the Northwest." www.cse.pdx.edu/wetlands/nwnutria .dir/nnwEI.htm.

Richardson, Scott. *East Bay Bird Guide*. Olympia, Wa.: Black Hills Audubon, 1997.

Rothenberg, David. *Why Birds Sing*. New York: Basic Books, 2005.

Sewall, Richard. *The Life of Emily Dickinson*. Cambridge, Mass.: Harvard University Press, 1974.

Sexton, Anne. "Her Kind." In *The Complete Poems*. Boston: Houghton Mifflin, 1981.

Sontag, Susan. "Regarding the Torture of Others." *New York Times*, May 23, 2004.

Thoreau, Henry David. *Walden*. 1854. New York: New American Library, 1960.

Thurman, Robert. *The Tibetan Book of the Dead*. New York: Bantam Books, 1994.

Tuttle, Merlin. *America's Neighborhood Bats: Understanding and Learning to Live in Harmony with Them*. Austin: University of Texas Press, 1988.

Welty, Joel. *The Life of Birds*. Philadelphia: Saunders, 1975.

Whitman, Walt. *Leaves of Grass*. Universal Library. New York: Grosset & Dunlap, n.d.

Willis, Patricia. "On 'An Octopus.'" www.english.uiuc.edu/maps/poets/m_r/moore/octopus.htm.

Wittgenstein, Ludwig. "The Inner and the Outer." In *Last Writings on the Philosophy of Psychology*. Ed. G. H. von Wright and Heikki Nyman. Trans. C. G. Luckhardt and Maximilian A. E. Aue. Vol. 2. Chicago: University of Chicago Press, 1982–92.

Wolf, Jaime. "Canceled Flight" (on the development of the jetpack). *New York Times*, June 11, 2000.